ANNUAL REVIEW OF GERONTOLOGY AND GERIATRICS

VOLUME 37, 2017

Editors

Annual Review of Gerontology and Geriatrics

Contemporary Issues and Future Directions in Lesbian, Gay, Bisexual, and Transgender Aging

VOLUME 37, 2017

Volume Editors

KRISTINA M. HASH, PhD, LICSW
ANISSA ROGERS, PhD, MSW, MA, LCSW

Series Editor

TONI C. ANTONUCCI, PhD

SPRINGER PUBLISHING COMPANY
NEW YORK

Springer Publishing Company, LLC
11 West 42nd Street
New York, NY 10036
www.springerpub.com

Acquisitions Editor: Sheri W. Sussman
Composition: Exeter Premedia Services Pvt. Ltd.

ISBN: 978-0-8261-2572-9
E-book ISBN: 978-0-8261-2573-6
ISSN: 0198-8794
Online ISSN: 1944-4036

17 18 19/ 5 4 3 2 1

Contents

About the Volume Editors

Kristina M. Hash, PhD, LICSW, is a professor in the School of Social Work and Director of the Gerontology Certificate Program at West Virginia University. She holds a PhD in social work from Virginia Commonwealth University, a Master of Social Work Degree and Graduate Gerontology Certificate from West Virginia University, and a Bachelor of Arts Degree from St. Catherine University. Her research interests include geriatric education, rural gerontology, LGBT issues, and the use of technology in teaching and research. Her work has been published in the *Journal of Gerontological Social Work, Journal of Gay and Lesbian Social Services, Clinical Social Work Journal*, and *Geriatric and Gerontology Education,* as well as in edited books. She is an editor and cowrote several chapters in *Aging in Rural Places: Programs, Policies, and Professional Practice* (Springer Publishing, 2015). She has taught courses on diversity, health and aging, rural gerontology, social work practice, social work research, and human behavior in the social environment.

Dr. Hash is an expert trainer and consultant for the Council on Social Work Education's National Center for Gerontological Social Work Education, was one of 15 participants chosen nationally for the National Institute of Aging First Annual Institute on Aging and Social Work, and has been an investigator for four geriatric education grants funded by the John A. Hartford Foundation and the Department of Health and Human Services/Health Resources and Services Administration/Bureau of Health Professions. She was a recipient of the Outstanding Principal Investigator Award from the New York Academy of Medicine's Social Work Leadership Institute, the David Z. Morgan Award for Excellence in Geriatric Education from the WV Geriatric Education Center and WV Geriatrics Society, and the Judith Gold Stitzel Award for teaching and leadership from the West Virginia University Center for Women's Studies.

Her practice background includes positions in home health care, social work continuing education, and research and program evaluation. Additionally, she has been involved in several volunteer activities with community-based agencies serving older adults. Her experience as a caregiver for her grandmother was the driving force behind her interest in social work and aging.

Anissa Rogers, PhD, MSW, MA, LCSW, is a professor of social work at the University of Portland in Portland, Oregon, where she has been teaching since 1999. She currently serves as the Director of the Social Work Program. She teaches courses across the social work curriculum as well as courses on gerontology, human sexuality, gender and the body, suffering and death, and international social work.

Dr. Rogers earned a bachelor's degree in psychology and MSW and PhD degrees in social work at the University of Utah. She also earned an MA degree in psychology at Ball State University. While working on her PhD, she earned a certificate in gerontology in which she specialized in mental health and aging. Dr. Rogers is also a licensed clinical social worker in the state of Oregon with an active private practice in animal assisted therapy with older adults and hospice patients.

While working on her PhD, Dr. Rogers worked with Utah state's Administration on Aging to develop mental health assessment tools for community-dwelling elders. In New Hampshire, she worked with the statewide Elder's Network to identify aging-related legislative priorities. More recently, Dr. Rogers has been developing gerontology-related placements and programs for undergraduate social work students. In addition, she has been involved in various community-based clinical and research projects with the older LGBT community in Portland and has written a textbook, Human Behavior in the Social Environment, which is in its fourth edition with Routledge Publishers. Dr. Rogers served on the board for Oregon's chapter of *National Association of Social Workers* (NASW), is a Hartford Faculty Scholar, and was the recipient of the Mit Joyner Gerontology Leadership Award in 2005. She also has been involved with various national organizations such as The Eldercare Workforce Alliance, the Gero-Ed Center, and the Association for Gerontology Education in Social Work.

Contributors

Jane Aronson, PhD, MSW, School of Social Work, McMaster University, Hamilton, ON

Shari Brotman, PhD, School of Social Work, McGill University, Montreal, QC

Sandra S. Butler, PhD, School of Social Work, University of Maine, Orono, ME

Andrea Daley, PhD, MSW, York University School of Social Work, Toronto, ON

Loralee Gillis, BA, Rainbow Health Ontario, Toronto, ON

Kristina M. Hash, PhD, LICSW, Professor, School of Social Work; Director, Gerontology Certificate Program, West Virginia University, Morgantown, West Virginia

Jennifer Hillman, PhD, Department of Psychology, Pennsylvania State University-Berks, Reading, PA

Shawn D. King, PhD, LISW-S, Private Practice, Athens, OH

Judith A. MacDonnell, PhD, MEd, RN, School of Nursing, York University, Toronto, ON

Mariann Mankowski, PhD, MSW, School of Social Work, West Virginia University, Morgantown, WV

Nancy A. Orel, PhD, LPC, College of Health and Human Services, Bowling Green State University, Bowling Green, OH

Virginia E. Richardson, PhD, College of Social Work, The Ohio State University, Columbus, OH

Anissa Rogers, PhD, MSW, MA, LCSW, Professor of social work, University of Portland, Portland, Oregon

Kristin S. Scherrer, PhD, LCSW, Department of Social Work, Metropolitan State University of Denver, Denver

Kenneth T. South, MDIV, American Academy of HIV Medicine, Washington, DC

Melissa St. Pierre, PhD, MA, York University, Toronto, ON

Tarynn M. Witten, PhD, LCSW, FGSA, Center for the Study of Biological Complexity, Virginia Commonwealth University, Richmond, VA

Previous Volumes in the Series

Vol. 36, 2016: Optimizing Physical Activity and Function Across All Settings

Editors: Barbara Resnick, PhD, CRNP, FGSA, FAANP, and Marie Boltz, PhD, RN, GNP-BC, FGSA, FAAN

Vol. 35, 2015: Subjective Aging: New Developments and Future Directions

Editors: Manfred Diehl, PhD, and Hans-Werner Wahl, PhD

Vol. 34, 2014: Genetics

Editor: Richard Sprott, PhD

Vol. 33, 2013: Healthy Longevity: A Global Approach

Editors: Jean-Marie Robine, DEA, DED, Carol Jagger, PhD, and Eileen M. Crimmins, PhD

Vol. 32, 2012: Emerging Perspectives on Resilience in Adulthood and Later Life

Editors: Bert Hayslip, Jr., PhD, and Gregory C. Smith, PhD

Vol. 31, 2011: Pathways Through Transitions of Care for Older Adults

Editors: Peggye Dilworth-Anderson, PhD, and Mary H. Palmer, PhD

Vol. 30, 2010: Biobehavioral Perspectives on Health in Later Life

Editor: Keith E. Whitfield, PhD

Vol. 29: Life-Course Perspectives on Late Life Health Inequalities

Editors: Toni C. Antonucci, PhD, and James S. Jackson, PhD

Vol. 28: Gerontological and Geriatric Education

Editors: Harvey L. Sterns, PhD, and Marie A. Bernard, MD

Vol. 27: Biopsychosocial Approaches to Longevity

Editors: Leonard W. Poon, PhD, DPhil, and Thomas T. Perls, MD, MPH

Vol. 26: The Crown of Life Dynamics of the Early Postretirement Period

Editors: Jacquelyn Boone James, PhD, and Paul Wink, PhD

Vol. 25: Aging Health Care Workforce Issues

Editors: Toni Miles, MD, PhD, and Antonio Furino, PhD, JD

Vol. 24: Focus on Intergenerational Relations Across Time and Place

Editors: Merril Silverstein, PhD, and K. Warner Schaie, PhD

Vol. 23: Focus on Aging in Context: Socio-Physical Environments

Editors: Hans Werner Wahl, PhD, Rick J. Scheidt, PhD, and Paul G. Windley, PhD

Vol. 22: Focus on Economic Outcomes in Later Life

Editors: Stephen Crystal, PhD, and Dennis Shea, PhD

Vol. 21: Focus on Modern Topics in the Biology of Aging

Editors: Vincent C. Cristofalo, PhD, and Richard Adelman, PhD

Vol. 20: Focus on the End of Life: Scientific and Social Issues

Editor: M. Powell Lawton, PhD

Preface

The past decade has seen significant progress in the recognition and rights of lesbian, gay, bisexual, and transgender (LGBT) persons of all ages. Changes in social attitudes about and policies affecting LGBT persons have helped to improve the mental, social, emotional, physical, spiritual, and economic health and well-being of LGBT individuals. These positive changes have had important implications for LGBT individuals as they age, who often face various challenges with health, caregiving, and living conditions. Research on older LGBT adults also has been increasing, highlighting the unique challenges those in this community face. Older cohorts of LGBT adults have experienced a lifetime of negative events and treatment, but they also have built resilience in the face of those experiences. While positive changes are occurring in societal attitudes about and treatment of older LGBT adults, more research is needed to better understand the challenges those in this community face that affect their health and well being as they age.

This volume brings together current research in health, policy, and psychosocial arenas important to older LGBT adults and offers recommendations on best practices and future directions for those working with this population. The volume is organized into three sections. The first section provides an introduction to the issues faced by older LGBT adults and provides context for the remaining chapters. The second section focuses on critical issues for older LGBT adults, with chapters on caregiving; mental health; social services; sexuality and sexual health; families and social supports; health and well-being for transgender and bisexual older adults; and special issues for older LGBT veterans and rural-dwelling older adults. The third section examines programs and policies for older LGBT adults and offers concluding comments for professionals working with older LGBT adults.

ANNUAL REVIEW OF GERONTOLOGY AND GERIATRICS

VOLUME 37, 2017

CHAPTER 1

Introduction to LGBT Aging

Kristina M. Hash and Anissa Rogers

ABSTRACT

This chapter provides an introduction to the volume, Contemporary Issues and Future Directions in Lesbian, Gay, Bisexual, and Transgender (LGBT) Aging. The volume examines current research, concepts, and theories related to the unique experience of aging as a sexual and gender minority. Issues such as caregiving, sexual health, social supports, and mental health among this population as well as the experiences of bisexual and transgender elders and those who are veterans and residents of rural communities are discussed within the volume. The larger issues of policies and services targeting the needs of older LGBT adults are also addressed. Future directions and opportunities to improve the aging experiences of this population are offered throughout the volume. This introductory chapter will set the stage for these topics and issues by providing a background to the field, the population, and the contemporary issues that impact their lives and well-being.

INTRODUCTION

June 26, 2013 marked a momentous event in U.S. history. The decision in the case of the *United States v. Windsor,* declared:

> Holding: Section 3 of the Defense of Marriage Act is unconstitutional as a deprivation of the equal liberty of persons that is protected by the Fifth Amendment. Judgment: Affirmed, 5–4 (www.scotusblog.com/case-files/cases/windsor-v-united-states-2)

http://dx.doi.org/10.1891/0198-8794.37.1

Two years after the Defense of Marriage Act (DOMA) was struck down, the U.S. Supreme Court legalized same-sex marriage across the United States. The plaintiff in the 2013 Supreme Court decision was Edith Windsor. Born in 1929, Windsor spent over 40 years with her same-sex partner, Thea Spyer. During their life together, they kept the nature of their relationship a secret from coworkers and employers. When Spyer was diagnosed with multiple sclerosis, Windsor eventually took an early retirement to care for her full time. Although they had been engaged since 1967, the couple was married legally in Canada in 2007. In addition to being married, the couple had drafted legal documents to ensure property rights and other inheritance for each other. When Spyer passed in 2009, Windsor was required to pay $363,053 in inheritance taxes to the Internal Revenue Service since their marriage was not legal in the United States. In response, Windsor filed a lawsuit in 2010 against the federal government (Gabbett, 2013). This suit and the 81-year-old widow led the way to legalized marriage for same-sex couples in the United States.

"Call me Caitlyn," appears on the cover of a magazine to promote a groundbreaking story and collection of photos in Vanity Fair. Born as Bruce Jenner, Caitlyn Jenner came out as transgender to the world in 2015 at the age of 65. Jenner was an American hero, winning a gold medal in the decathlon in the 1976 Olympics, but since a child felt as though she was trapped in the wrong body. Delighted to become her true self, her first tweet on Twitter as Caitlyn announced, "Welcome to the world Caitlyn. Can't wait for you to get to know her/me." She gained four million followers on Twitter that day (Bissinger, 2015).

The recent events centered around Edith Windsor and Caitlyn Jenner reflect a movement in attitudes and policy in support of gay, lesbian, bisexual, and transgender individuals in the United States as well as abroad. As impactful as their stories have been, they in many ways mirror the life experiences of many older gay, lesbian, bisexual, and transgender persons who have not received the same public attention. This chapter will provide a foundation for understanding these experiences and serve as an introduction to chapters that will detail current research on critical topics regarding and future directions for better understanding and supporting older LGBT adults. As such, it will offer a context from which to understand the lives of older LGBT adults, including important terms related to the population, the historic times in which they have lived and public opinion surrounding them, the basics of LGBT aging, and theories that are useful for understanding their experiences. The chapter will conclude with an overview of the volume and an invitation to the reader to explore its knowledge and vision.

IMPORTANT TERMS RELATED TO THE POPULATION

As with describing all minority populations, terminology and language matter. The focus of this volume will be on older gay male, lesbian, bisexual, and transgender persons. It is assumed that "older" will identify individuals 65 years of age and older. Although it is debatable whether this is truly the marker of when a person is "old," it is an age that is commonly used in research and in major reports such as Healthy People 2020 (U.S. Department of Health and Human Services [USDHHS], 2010). Many would also question whether the designation of LGBT is inclusive enough given the complexity of gender identity and sexual orientation. In fact, the initials "Q" for queer or questioning and "I" for intersex are often included in the group identifier (LGBTQI). This volume, however, will primarily align with the majority of research in this area and the identifiers L, G, B, and T. In general, the following definitions provided by the Human Rights Campaign (n.d.) will apply:

Lesbian: A woman who is emotionally, romantically or sexually attracted to other women.

Gay: A person who is emotionally, romantically or sexually attracted to members of the same gender

Bisexual: A person emotionally, romantically or sexually attracted to more than one sex, gender or gender identity though not necessarily simultaneously, in the same way or to the same degree

Transgender: An umbrella term for people whose gender identity and/or expression is different from cultural expectations based on the sex they were assigned at birth.

HISTORIC TIMES AND PUBLIC OPINION

Although Edith Windsor and Caitlyn Jenner have a few decades difference in age, they and other older LGBT adults have lived primarily through times that have been less than supportive of their sexual orientations and gender identities. Individuals who are currently 65+ would have lived through times when there were laws against homosexuality and diagnoses from the psychiatric community to negatively label homosexual and transgender persons. In fact, it was not until 1973 that the American Psychological Association (APA) removed "homosexuality" from its diagnostic manual for mental illnesses. Transgender identity is still included as a condition in the manual and is designated as "Gender Dysphoria." Antisodomy laws, removal of homosexuals from federal jobs and the military, and police harassment of the patrons of gay bars became commonplace during the 1930s–1960s. The 1980s and the AIDS epidemic saw a growing fear and hatred of gay men in particular. Beginning in the 1990s, a number of states enacted amendments to their constitutions defining marriage only between a man and a woman. At the federal level, this definition was solidified by the DOMA, passed by Congress in 1996 (Eaklor, 2011; Faderman, 2015).

The lives of older LGBT adults have also been influenced by positive events. The 1930s saw the openings of gay bars and LGBT advocacy groups and societies began forming in the 1950s and 1960s. The Kinsey Report (1953) supported diversity in sexual orientation and behavior and as mentioned, the APA removed homosexuality from its list of mental disorders in 1973. In addition, a major event occurred in 1969 in the Greenwich Village section of New York City. The "Stonewall Rebellion" was a several days long protest by large numbers of LGBT persons in response to decades of harassment this population faced in gay bars. This rebellion marked the start of the Gay Rights Movement. Other steps forward include positive changes beginning in the 1990s, including a number of states and municipalities that passed policies to ensure equity for LGBT persons and their relationships. This, of course, eventually led to the repeal of DOMA and passing of same-sex marriage rights nationwide. As examples of other positive events at the national level, a hate crimes law was passed in 2009 that included LGBT individuals and the Don't Ask Don't Tell in the military policy was struck down in 2011. Despite these moves forward, there is still much work to do on behalf of LGBT persons of all ages. For example, at the time of this publication, there is still no federal law protecting LGBT individuals in the workplace or in housing, and there are movements to repeal same-sex marriage (Eaklor, 2011; Faderman, 2015).

Public opinion has also shifted in a positive direction with regard to sexual orientation and gender identity. The Williams Institute (Flores, 2014) conducted a review of 325 public opinion surveys between 1977 and 2014 related to this population. Results suggest that public support for gay men and lesbians in the past 30 years has doubled. Far fewer polls have sought opinions about transgender persons but according to those that have, there has been a 40% increase in favorable opinion toward this population between 2005 and 2011. Surveys regarding bisexual persons are also few in number but in 2011 surveys showed more favorable opinions as opposed to less favorable toward this population. Not surprisingly, support for marriage equality increased steadily between the 1980s and 2000s. Currently, over 70% of those polled believe that there should be protections for LGBT persons in the workplace.

THE BASICS OF LGBT AGING

LGBT individuals experience many of the same challenges in aging as their non-LGBT counterparts. Older adults, in general, experience increased chronic health conditions and disability. This often results in difficulty with activities of daily living and instrumental activities of daily living and need for some form of assistance or care. Although not a normal part of aging, conditions such as Alzheimer's disease and related dementias also increase with advancing age (Berlau, Corrada, Peltz, & Kawas, 2012; Centers for Disease Control and Prevention, 2013; Corrada, Brookmeyer, Paganini-Hill, Berlau, & Kawas, 2010). Many older adults also take on roles such as retiree, grandparent, or caregiver. Chronic illness, caregiving, and financial concerns are also common experiences of older adults (National Institute on Aging & USDHHS, 2007; Thiele & Whelan, 2006). Research has shown that older LGBT adults face issues such as those mentioned above as well as additional challenges as they age. In terms of health conditions, this population experiences higher rates of obesity, disability, and HIV (Fredriksen-Goldsen et al., 2011). Related to mental health, they have been thought to be at greater risk for depression, suicide, loneliness, violence, and substance abuse (Fredriksen-Goldsen et al., 2011). Abuse and violence can be lifelong experiences and can contribute to health and mental health problems for those in this population (Fredriksen-Goldsen et al., 2011; Kidd & Witten, 2008; Morrow, 2001). Long-term discrimination, fear, and the need to hide their true selves have added to their poorer health and mental health outcomes as well. This treatment and fear have also caused older members of this population to be apprehensive about seeking formal health and social services, such as in-home care, support groups, adult day care, case management, mental health services, and skilled nursing care (Cahill & South, 2002; Gugliucci, Weaver, Kimmel, Littlefield, Hollander, & Hennessy, 2013; Hash, 2006; McFarland & Sanders, 2003; Stein, Beckerman, & Sherman, 2010). In terms of receiving skilled nursing care in a long-term care or assisted living facilities, older LGBT adults are particularly concerned about separation from partners, conjugal visits, sharing rooms with non-LGBT persons, and unsupportive behaviors from residents and staff (Gugliucci et al., 2013; Stein, Beckerman, & Sherman, 2010).

Clearly, the striking down of the DOMA and the federal enactment of marriage equality in the United States have been the most important policy advances to date for LGBT persons of all ages. As mentioned, a policy at the federal level protecting LGBT individuals in the workplace has not been enacted at the time of this publication. This means that members of this population can be fired or passed over for hiring or promotion because of their sexual orientation or gender identity. Likewise, LGBT persons can still be discriminated against in terms of access to housing as legal protections do not universally exist in this realm for this population. It is important to understand that even with the policy advancements and protections, older LGBT adults have spent the majority of their lives in the absence of equal rights and have endured negative attitudes and treatment from society as well as from professionals and those close to them.

When considering the impact of public opinion and policies, it is also critical to understand that when talking about older LGBT adults, different age cohorts are included. As such, older LGBT individuals have lived in similar yet different times depending on when they were born and the ages in which they experienced events and changes. In addition to cohort differences, the influence of geography should also be acknowledged. For example, gender and sexual minorities residing in small towns and rural areas may not have had access to more welcoming communities that larger cities enjoy. Other factors such as gender, ethnicity, and socioeconomic status can also affect the experiences of LGBT persons throughout the life course.

THEORIES FOR UNDERSTANDING LGBT AGING

Understanding the unique experiences of older LGBT adults can and has been accomplished by applying a variety of theories to their experiences. The theory of intersectionality and the minority stress perspective are two that are very applicable and are utilized by chapters in this volume. As mentioned above, cohort and other differences can impact the experiences of older LGBT adults. The theory of intersectionality is useful for looking at persons based upon differences and the layering or intersections of their various statuses. For example, an older lesbian of color would have unique experiences and challenges based upon these three identities. Using this theory, the diversity that exists within the older LGBT population can be identified and considered. Older persons are more different from each other than they are similar, by the simple fact that they have had sixty or more years to build varying experiences. Adding to age, the characteristics of class, gender, ethnicity, education, religion, ability/disability, geographic location, and gender identity and sexual orientation increase this diversity (Hash & Weirich, in press). Unfortunately, few studies have examined the experiences of diverse older LGBT adults.

The U.S. population, in general, is becoming more ethnically diverse, and the proportion of ethnic minorities compared to other elders has grown from 17% in 2003 to 21% in 2014 and will rise to 29% by 2030 (Administration on Aging [AOA], 2014). Unfortunately, we know very little about older LGBT adults of color, as the literature has largely not reflected their experiences or participation in research (Fredriksen-Goldsen & Muraco, 2010). Fredriksen-Golsen et al. (2011) conducted the largest and most ethnically diverse study to date on older LGBT adults. Experiences of ethnically diverse older LGBT adults revealed differences in "disclosure, social support and religious and spiritual activities among LGBT older adult participants as differentiated by race and ethnicity" (p. 18). Specifically, as compared to their older White counterparts, Asian/Pacific Islander LGBT adults had lower levels of disclosure and Hispanics had lower levels of social support. In addition, African Americans and Native Americans in their study were more likely to engage in religious or spiritual activities.

Although considered a social minority, older women of all orientations are the majority in number. The ratio of women to men who are 65+ in the United States is 129 women for every 100 men. The ratio is even higher in later years: for ages 85+, there are 200 women for every 100 men (AOA, 2014). Older lesbians have also been found to experience more unique challenges in aging than their gay male counterparts. In particular, women have been found to have lower incomes. However, women may be more likely to have partners, larger social support networks, and housing companions than men (Fredriksen-Goldsen & Muraco, 2010). Similarly, older LGBT adults who live in rural communities can also be viewed as social minorities with unique experiences as they age. Although few studies have focused on this population, what is known is that they often have the challenge of being isolated from specialized services and supports for LGBT persons that often exist in larger areas. They may also experience increased homophobia in their communities and be more reluctant to come out to professionals, family, and others (Comerford, Henson-Stroud, Sionainn, & Wheeler; 2004; King & Dabelko-Schoeny, 2009; Lee & Quam, 2013; Oswald & Culton, 2003).

The minority stress perspective may also be used to view the experiences of this population. This model views LGBT persons of all ages as social minorities, or members of a group who are considered inferior to or "less than" the majority (non-LGBT persons; Meyer, 2003; Mink, Lindley, & Weinstein, 2014). As such, members of this population often experience chronic, excess stress related to the stigma, prejudice, and discrimination faced throughout their lives. This stress can put LGBT individuals at greater risk for mental and physical health problems (Frost, Lehavot, & Meyer, 2015; Institute of Medicine, 2011; Meyer, 2003; Mink, Lindley, & Weinstein, 2014). Additional stressors related to other minority statuses may also be involved, such as gender, ethnicity, and socioeconomic status. However, in response to this treatment, individuals may build resilience, coping mechanisms, and social supports. Similarly, the LGBT community as a whole may also come together to combat such conditions through what is called minority coping. Positively identifying with a minority status can also serve as a mediator of stress for individuals (Meyer, 2003).

In addition to theories, competencies and guidelines have been developed to assist professionals working with older LGBT adults. The Partnership for Health in Aging (2010) has developed multidisciplinary competencies for health professionals related to the care of older adults of all orientations and identities.

Other professional organizations have drafted competencies for specific disciplines such as social work (e.g., Social Work Leadership Institute & the Council on Social Work Education, n.d.). Given the unique issues faced by LGBT elders, practice guidelines and competencies have also been put forward to ensure that their care is competent and sensitive. In 2012, the APA published the Guidelines for Psychological Practice with Lesbian, Gay, and Bisexual Clients (APA, 2012) for clients of all ages. Specific to older LGBT adults, the guidelines insist that practitioners acknowledge the historical period in which persons have lived, the age and social times in which they "came out," and the societal attitudes and policies that have impacted their lives. The APA also stresses the importance of multiple minority statuses (age, gender, ethnicity, and disability) and their effect on the lives of LGBT persons. Following these guidelines, practitioners can assist LGBT elders employ coping mechanisms that they have built throughout their lives to help them manage the challenges presented in aging and deal with continued oppression related to being LGBT (APA, 2012; Hash & Rogers, 2013). Fredriksen-Goldsen et al. (2014) integrated the Geriatric Social Work Competencies (Social Work Leadership Institute & the Council on Social Work Education, n.d.) into what is known from research about sexual and gender minority elders and developed 10 competencies for working with and developing programs for LGBT older adults. Among other skills and actions, the competencies challenge social work professionals to examine their own attitudes toward the population; consider oppressive factors in the larger social environment including policies; identify additional minority statuses affecting individuals; and apply appropriate theories and current research to practice.

Building on the competencies mentioned above, Crisp, Wayland, and Gordon (2008) propose a model for social work and related practice with LGBT elders. The "age competent and gay affirmative practice" (p. 6) model combines culturally competent knowledge, attitudes, and skills for work with LGBT individuals with the geriatric social work competencies. This approach focuses on and builds upon the strengths and resiliency of LGBT elders. Similarly, Hash and Rogers (2013) advocate for an approach to clinical mental health practice with this population that can be applied to the work of other disciplines:

> Competent and effective practice with older LGBT elders begins with an understanding of normative aging issues as well as the unique challenges faced by this population. The awareness of the strengths they have built throughout their lifetime to overcome barriers to their health and happiness is also essential. This understanding provides a foundation from which to identify appropriate theories and models of intervention for working with individual clients. (p. 256)

CONCLUSION AND INVITATION TO THE READER

Due to the sweeping changes in policies and public opinion, recent years will mark a historic and exciting point in time for the older LGBT population and their allies. The editors and authors of this volume would like to extend an invitation to the readers to expand their knowledge on the many issues impacting this population and discover possibilities for continuing improvement for the lives and well-being of this special population of older adults. Students, professionals, educators, policy makers, and others should find the content to be very timely and applicable to clinical practice as well as work with policy and programming to support this population. This volume will examine the contemporary issues facing LGBT elders. Chapters include up-to-date research and theory on issues such as sexual health, caregiving, and mental health for older members of this population as well as their families and support systems. The unique experiences of bisexual and transgender elders and veterans and rural residents will also be considered. The challenges of providing health and social services and the impact of public and health policy on this population will also be addressed. Each of these chapters will cover a background and definitions of key concepts, a summary of current research on the topic, and the trends and future directions related to the specific issue for this population. A concluding chapter will follow to summarize the current research and progress that has been made on behalf of older LGBT adults as well as propose advancements in research, policy, and practice to ensure the continued movement toward positive and productive aging for this population.

REFERENCES

Administration on Aging. (2014). *A profile of older Americans: 2014*. Washington, DC: United States Department of Health and Human Services, Administration on Aging, Administration for Community Living. Retrieved from http://www.aoa.gov/Aging_Statistics/Profile/2014/docs/2014-Profile.pdf

American Psychological Association (APA). (2012). Guidelines for psychological practice with lesbian, gay, and bisexual clients. *American Psychologist, 67*, 10–42.

Berlau, D. J., Corrada, M. M., Peltz, C. R., & Kawas, C. H. (2012). Disability in the oldest-old: Incidence and risk factors in the 90+ Study. *American Journal of Geriatric Psychiatry, 20*(2), 159–168.

Bissinger, B. (2015, June 30). Caitlyn Jenner: The full story. *Vanity Fair*. Retrieved from http://www.vanityfair.com/hollywood/2015/06/caitlyn-jenner-bruce-cover-annie-leibovitz

Cahill, S., & South, K. (2002). Policy issues affecting lesbian, gay, bisexual, and transgender people in retirement. *Generations, 26*(2), 49–54.

Centers for Disease Control and Prevention. (2013). *The state of aging and health in America 2013*. Atlanta, GA: Centers for Disease Control and Prevention, US Department of Health and Human Services. Retrieved from http://www.cdc.gov/aging/pdf/state-aging-health-in-america-2013.pdf

Comerford, S. A., Henson-Stroud, M., Sionainn, C., & Wheeler, E. (2004). Crone songs: Voices of lesbian elders on aging in a rural environment. *Affilia, 19*(4), 418–436.

Corrada, M. M., Brookmeyer, R., Paganini-Hill, A., Berlau, D., & Kawas, C. H. (2010), Dementia incidence continues to increase with age in the oldest old: The 90+ study. *Annals of Neurology, 67*, 114–121.

Crisp, C., Wayland, S., & Gordon, T. (2008). Older gay, lesbian, and bisexual adults: Tools for age-competent and gay affirmative practice. *Journal of Gay and Lesbian Social Services, 20*(1–2), 5–29.

Eaklor, V. L. (2011). *Queer America: A people's GLBT history of the United States*. New York, NY: The New Press.

Faderman, L. (2015). *The gay revolution: The story of struggle*. New York, NY: Simon and Schuster.

Flores, A. R. (2014). National trends in public opinion on LGBT rights in the United States. *The Williams Institute*. Retrieved from http://williamsinstitute.law.ucla.edu/wp-content/uploads/POP-natl-trends-nov-2014.pdf

Fredriksen-Goldsen, K. I., Kim, H. J., Emlet, C. A., Muraco, A., Erosheva, E. A., Hoy-Ellis, C. P., et al. (2011). *The aging and health report: Disparities and resilience among lesbian, gay, bisexual, and transgender older adults*. Seattle, WA: Institute for Multigenerational Health.

Fredriksen-Goldsen, K. I., Hoy-Ellis, C. P., Goldsen, J., Emlet, C. A., & Hooyman, N. R. (2014). Creating a vision for the future: Key competencies and strategies for culturally competent practice with lesbian, gay, bisexual, and transgender (LGBT) older adults in the health and human services. *Journal of Gerontological Social Work, 57*(2–4), 80–107.

Fredriksen-Goldsen, K. I., & Muraco, A. (2010). Aging and sexual orientation: A 25-year review of the literature. *Research on Aging, 32*(3), 372–413.

Frost, D. M., Lehavot, K., & Meyer, I. H. (2015). Minority stress and physical health among sexual minority individuals. *Journal of Behavioral Medicine, 38*(1), 1–8.

Gabbett, A. (2013, June 26). Edith Windsor and Thea Spyer: 'A love affair that just kept on and on and on.' *The Guardian*. Retrieved from http://www.theguardian.com/world/2013/jun/26/edith-windsor-thea-spyer-doma

Gugliucci, M. R., Weaver, S. A., Kimmel, D. C, Littlefield, M., Hollander, L., & Hennessy, J. (2013). *Gay, lesbian, bisexual, and transgender (GLBT) aging in Maine: Community needs assessment* Portland, ME: AARP. Retrieved from http://sagemaine.org/needs-assessment.html

Hash, K. M. (2006). Caregiving and post-caregiving experiences of midlife and older gay men and lesbians. *Journal of Gerontological Social Work, 47*(3/4), 121–138.

Hash, K. M., & Rogers, A. (2013). Clinical practice with older LGBT clients: Overcoming lifelong stigma through strength and resilience. *Clinical Social Work Journal, 41*(3), 249–257.

Hash, K. M., & Weirich, M. R. (in press). Aging. In E. Fullmer & N. A. Newfield (Eds.), *Connecting the dots, intersectionality and cultural intelligence: A guide for professionals.* Dubuque, IA: Kendall Hunt.

Human Rights Campaign. (n.d.). *Glossary of terms.* Retrieved from http://www.hrc.org/resources/glossary-of-terms

Institute of Medicine. (2011). *The health of lesbian, gay, bisexual, and transgender people: Building a foundation for better understanding.* Washington, DC: The National Academies Press. Retrieved from http://www.ncbi.nlm.nih.gov/books/NBK64806

Kidd, J. D., & Witten, T. M. (2008). Understanding spirituality and religiosity in the transgender community: Implications for aging. *Journal of Religion, Spirituality and Aging, 20*(1–2), 29–62.

King, S., & Dabelko-Schoeny, H. (2009). "Quite frankly, I have doubts about remaining": Aging-in-place and health care access for rural midlife and older lesbian, gay, and bisexual individuals. *Journal of LGBT Health Research, 5*(1/2), 10–21.

Lee, M. G., & Quam, J. K. (2013). Comparing supports for LGBT aging in rural versus urban areas. *Journal of Gerontological Social Work, 56*(2), 112–126.

McFarland, P. L., & Sanders, S. (2003). Pilot study about the needs of older gays and lesbians: What social workers need to know. *Journal of Gerontological Social Work, 40*(3), 67–80.

Meyer, I. H. (2003). Prejudice, social stress, and mental health in lesbian, gay, and bisexual populations: Conceptual issues and research evidence. *Psychological Bulletin, 129*(5), 674–697.

Mink, M. D., Lindley, L. L., & Weinstein, A. A. (2014). Stress, stigma, and sexual minority status: The intersectional ecology model of LGBTQ health. *Journal of Gay and Lesbian Social Services, 26*(4), 502–521.

Morrow, D. F. (2001). Older gays and lesbians: Surviving a generation of hate and violence. *Journal of Gay and Lesbian Social Services, 13*(1–2), 151–169.

National Institute on Aging & U.S. Department of Health and Human Services (USDHHS). (2007). *Growing Older in America: The health and retirement study.* Washington, DC: Author.

Oswald, R., & Culton, L. (2003). Under the rainbow: Rural gay life and its relevance for family providers. *Family Relations, 52*(1), 72–81.

Partnership for Health in Aging. (2010). *Multidisciplinary competencies in the care of older adults at the completion of the entry-level health professional degrees.* Retrieved from http://www.americangeriatrics.org/files/documents/health_care_pros/PHA_Multidisc_Competencies.pdf

Social Work Leadership Institute & the Council on Social Work Education. (n.d.). *Geriatric social work competency scale II with life long leadership skills.* Retrieved from http://www.cswe.org/File.aspx?id=25445

Stein, G., Beckerman, N., & Sherman, P. (2010). Lesbian and gay elders and long-term care: Identifying the unique psychosocial perspectives and challenges. *Journal of Gerontological Social Work, 53*(5), 421–435.

Thiele, D. M., & Whelan, T. A. (2006). Nature and dimensions of the grandparent role. *Marriage and Family Review*, *40*(1), 93–108.

U.S. Department of Health and Human Services (USDHHS). (2010). *Healthy People 2020*. Washington, DC: U.S. Department of Health and Human Services, Office of Disease Prevention and Health Promotion. Retrieved from https://www.healthypeople.gov

CHAPTER 2

The Sexuality and Sexual Health of LGBT Elders

Jennifer Hillman

ABSTRACT

Sexuality and sexual health represent lifelong needs that cut across sexual orientation, gender identity, and age. The goal of this chapter is to celebrate and address the diversity of sexuality and sexual health among older lesbian, gay, bisexual, and transgender (LGBT) adults. Key concepts including sexuality, sexual health, and older adulthood are defined, and age-normative changes and common forms of sexual dysfunction (e.g., vaginal dryness and erectile dysfunction) are identified. Their experience with health disparities are also addressed, including a lack of insurance coverage, insufficient numbers of culturally competent providers, and negative experiences with health care providers. Attention also will be given to LGBT elders' unique risk factors for HIV/AIDS, breast, cervical, prostate, and anal cancers. The chapter concludes with LGBT-affirming recommendations for both public policy and care providers.

BACKGROUND AND KEY CONCEPTS

Throughout this chapter on sexuality and sexual health, the umbrella term LGBT will be used in a purposeful attempt to acknowledge and include a variety of subpopulations. As used here, LGBT is intended to include individuals who may identify themselves as lesbian, gay, bisexual, transgender, intersex, two-spirit, queer, questioning, on the down low, men who love men, or women who love

http://dx.doi.org/10.1891/0198-8794.37.13

women. However, as important as it is to promote inclusiveness, it remains essential to recognize that individual LGBT populations remain unique and distinct from one another (Institute of Medicine, 2011). It is also important to remind anyone unfamiliar with LGBT issues that individuals who identify as transgender do so in terms of gender identity; their sexual orientation may be lesbian, gay, or bisexual. Sexuality will be defined broadly as one's sexual orientation, behavior, satisfaction, health, and dysfunction.

Factors that influence LGBT elders' sexuality and sexual health include culture, religion, spirituality, exposure to the media, health and human service systems (e.g., Fredriksen-Goldsen, Hoy-Ellis, Goldsen, Emlet, & Hooyman, 2014), ethnicity, urbanity, and age cohort (i.e., younger baby boomers vs. the oldest old; Hillman, 2012). For example, the influence of discrimination is particularly salient for LGBT elders over the age of 80, and it affects their physical and mental-health-related quality of life more negatively than it does for both middle-aged and older LGBT adults between the ages of 65 and 79. Further, oldest-old LGBT are significantly less likely to disclose their sexual orientation or any history of discrimination (e.g., physical, psychological, or sexual abuse) to a care provider, and are less likely to receive appropriate assessment or treatment (Fredriksen-Goldsen, Kim, Shiu, Goldsen, & Emlet, 2015). African American LGBT elders typically face not only ageism and heterosexism like their White LGBT peers, but also additional, synergistic challenges related to racism. Compared to their urban peers, research also suggests that rural LGBT elders are more likely to have lower household income and are less likely to disclose their sexual orientation to others, including their friends and siblings (Lee & Quam, 2013).

Significant gaps exist in the literature regarding LGBT elders' sexuality and sexual health. Most surveys focus upon the sexual activity of gay and lesbian elders; no national surveys are available to provide detailed information about the sexual activity of older bisexual and transgender adults. Most surveys also only focus upon sexual activity rather than more global measures of sexual health and satisfaction. The limited research findings available are often generated via convenience samples of predominantly White, well-educated participants (e.g., Averett, Yoon, & Jenkins, 2012). A lack of standardized self-identifiers also makes it difficult to gather accurate estimates of LGBT elders' sexual activity and health. For example, although transgender elders are often classified as female-to-male (FTM) or male-to-female (MTF) in research, they may self-report as postoperative, trans, intersex, butch woman, feminine man, or simply as male or female as per their identified or postoperative gender. Other factors make it difficult to obtain information specific to older LGBT adults. For example, although the age of 65 is typically used as the cutoff to define older adulthood, the Centers for Disease Control and Prevention (CDC) only provides information about HIV/AIDS among adults aged 50 and older. These discrepancies in recruiting, self-identification, and age cohorts can make it difficult to interpret and generalize many studies' findings.

Findings from large-scale national studies, including the National Social Life, Health, and Aging Project (NSHAP; Waite, Laumann, Das, & Schum, 2009), suggest that many men and women of all orientations engage in vaginal sex, oral sex, and masturbation well into their 80s and 90s. Additional findings from the NSHAP revealed that approximately 40% of women and 67% of men aged 65–74 engaged in "any [type] of sex" within the past year, compared to 17% of women and 39% of men aged 75–84 in the past year. Sexual activity also occurs within the context of disability and dementia, even in advanced age (Hillman, 2012).

Menopause, adrenopause, chronic and acute illness, and prescription and over-the-counter (OTC) medications can all contribute to the most common forms of sexual dysfunction in women (i.e., lack of sexual interest and vaginal dryness) and ED in men. Vaginal dryness and pain during intercourse affect approximately 40% of women over the age of 50; the incidence generally does not increase with age. In contrast, the older the man, the more likely he is to report ED. On average, nearly one-third of men aged 57–64 and nearly half of men aged 65–74 and 75–85 report experiencing ED (Waite et al., 2009). It is also important to note that most definitions of ED only consider the ability to engage in penetrative vaginal intercourse.

SEXUAL ACTIVITY OF LGBT ELDERS

The available research regarding the sexuality of older lesbians, typically defined as age 50 and older, suggests that the vast majority (80%) feel very positive about being a lesbian. An online survey of more than 450 self-identified, community-living lesbians over the age of 50 revealed that fewer than 15% had their first female-to-female sexual experience after they were 40 years of age (Averett et al., 2012). In terms of placing importance upon sex, only 22% of these older lesbians reported that sex per se was "very important" to them. Older lesbians also tend to place greater focus upon sexual and relationship satisfaction than the actual appearance of their bodies (Averett et al., 2012).

Information about sexual activity and satisfaction among older gay men is based primarily upon studies from the 1990s and earlier. Unfortunately, most of the current large-scale, national surveys of sexual activity (e.g., the NSHAP; Waite et al., 2009) fail to gather information about anal sex. The limited data available suggests that gay men over the age of 50 engage in sexual activity less frequently than their younger peers, but that their level of sexual satisfaction remains generally consistent. Although myths persist that older adults avoid the

Internet, studies also suggest that more than half of older gay men prefer to seek their partners online (Bolding, Davis, Sherr, Hart, & Elford, 2004).

Very limited data exists regarding the sexual activity and satisfaction of bisexual elders. Older bisexuals often appear "invisible" in research because they may identify as gay, lesbian, or heterosexual based upon the gender of their last partner. Available findings generally dispel the myth that bisexual elders are more promiscuous than their lesbian, gay, or heterosexual peers (e.g., Lovejoy et al., 2008). An additional challenge for bisexual elders is the distrust they may face from heterosexual and LG peers who assert that they choose a male or female partner out of convenience, or that they select an opposite-sex partner to better "pass" among heterosexuals (Israel & Mohr, 2004).

Research regarding the sexual activity of transgender elders attests to the diversity of this population. In one of the few existing studies, Cook-Daniels and Munson (2010) gathered responses from nearly 300 transgender adults over the age of 50. The sexual orientation of the participants ranged from lesbian (15%), gay (8%), bisexual (23%), heterosexual (17%), queer (12%), asexual/celibate (9%), to questioning (7%). More than half (54%) stated that either their own or their partner's sexual orientation changed at some point during their relationship. More than half (57%) of the transgender elders reported that they engaged in oral sex, and more than one third (37%) engaged in anal sex. Participation in sexual activity was influenced by personal likes and dislikes, pain and discomfort (e.g., FTM individuals taking testosterone may find vaginal penetration painful), religious beliefs, history of sexual trauma, and gender identity (e.g., consistent with their identified gender, some FTM participants used a dildo or prosthesis and avoided vaginal penetration). It was unclear what percentage of the total sample completed sex reassignment surgery; 40% of the respondents used clothing during sex to cover parts of their body inconsistent with their gender identity.

A rare survey of transgender adults who completed sex reassignment surgery (Cuypere et al., 2005) revealed that the procedure successfully met most of the participants' emotional and sexual expectations. FTM participants reported more powerful orgasms, and MTF participants reported more intense, longer orgasms. Some complications arose in which FTM elders experienced pain when using an erectile prosthesis, and some FTM elders experienced briefer orgasm. It is also important to note that this sample of transgender adults had the financial resources to undergo reassignment surgery.

Unfortunately, health disparities play a significant role in shaping LGBT elders' sexual health. Findings from national surveys reveal that fewer than one in four LGBT elders disclose their sexual orientation to a health care provider (Gelo, 2008), and that one in five LGBT baby boomers express little or no confidence that a health care provider will treat them with dignity or respect (MetLife, 2010). Concealing one's sexual identity from providers can lead to ineffective or injurious health care (Fassinger & Arseneau, 2007). Older adults in general report low rates of discussing sex with their health care provider (e.g., 22% of women and 38% of men over the age of 50; Lindau et al., 2007), and fear of discrimination makes it even less likely that LGBT elders will have that discussion with their care provider.

More than 40% of LGBT adults aged 50 and older suffer from at least one disability or chronic illness, and they are more likely to smoke, engage in binge drinking, have higher rates of heart disease and diabetes, and delay treatment-seeking behavior when compared to their heterosexual peers. Nearly one in three older LGBT adults report that they are depressed, and more than half report that they feel socially isolated and lonely (Fredriksen-Goldsen et al., 2011); LGBT minority elders may be at even greater risk (Fredriksen-Goldsen, Kim, Barkan, Muraco, & Hoy-Ellis, 2013). Additional disparities include a lack of insurance coverage, insufficient numbers of culturally competent providers, and negative experiences with health care providers. All of these aforementioned inequalities can work synergistically, and may place LGBT elders at greater risk for high-risk behaviors (e.g., having sex while under the influence of alcohol or other substances) and a lack of appropriate screening and treatment for sexual health care. A lack of *National Institutes of Health* (NIH) funding in LGBT-related health care research in areas other than HIV/AIDS provides evidence of additional disparity (Voyles, 2015). It is as though the U.S. government itself does not place value upon LGBT elders' overall sexual health and satisfaction.

OLDER LESBIANS AND BISEXUAL WOMEN

It is essential to acknowledge that LGBT elders represent four very different, subpopulations. In this section, unique issues in sexual health related to older LGBT elders are reviewed. For example, despite the prevalent myth held by both lesbians and their care providers that lesbians are not at risk for sexually transmitted diseases (STDs; McIntyre, Szewchuk, & Munro, 2010), evidence reveals that lesbian elders are not immune to the transmission of STDs. Nearly 50% of older lesbians report having heterosexual vaginal or anal intercourse at some point in their lives, and 20% of all women who never had heterosexual intercourse are infected with *human papillomavirus* (HPV) virus, the primary cause of cervical cancer. Although uncommon, female-to-female transmission of HIV (Hughes & Evans, 2003) and HPV are possible (Tracy, Schluterman, & Greenberg, 2013). It is important to remember that lesbians can transmit a variety of STDs via contact between skin, mucus membranes, and vaginal fluids. Accordingly, older lesbians and bisexual women should receive both routine STD screenings (e.g., pap smears) and appropriate preventative care messages (Addis, Mavies, Greene, MacBride-Stewart, & Shepherd, 2009).

Older lesbians face significant risk factors for cervical cancer including increased rates of smoking and obesity, and a lack of health insurance. Unfortunately, estimates suggest that only 50% of lesbians engage in routine pap testing, while more than 75% of their heterosexual female peers engage in routine testing. Failure to disclose one's sexual orientation, limited knowledge of HPV, lack of physician referral, and inaccurate physician advice all predicted low levels of screening (McIntyre et al., 2010; Tracy et al., 2013). Older lesbians also have a significantly higher 5-year and lifetime risk for developing breast cancer when compared to older heterosexual women. Risk factors for breast cancer among lesbians include lower numbers of pregnancies, births, abortions, and miscarriages, less frequent use of the birth control pill, a greater number of breast biopsies, and lower rates of insurance (Dibble, Roberts, & Nussey, 2004).

It is difficult to estimate the number of older bisexual women living with HIV/AIDS as the CDC does not include this category in their surveillance data. What is clear, however, is that any postmenopausal woman can find herself at increased risk of HIV infection. Thinning of the vaginal wall is more likely to provide micro- and macroscopic tears during sexual activity, allowing for easier access of HIV into the bloodstream. Overall reductions in immune system functioning also make it more likely for older women to contract the HIV virus, per exposure, when compared to their younger counterparts. Older lesbian and bisexual women are also less likely to have experience with condoms and are more likely to view them as a needless method of preventing pregnancy. Incorrect beliefs that HIV/AIDS affects only young gay men or drug users also make it unlikely that older lesbians and bisexual women will engage in HIV prevention or testing (see Hillman, 2012).

OLDER GAY AND BISEXUAL MEN

Gay and bisexual male elders also face unique challenges in relation to health disparities. Although more than 15% of new HIV/AIDS cases were among adults over the age of 50 in 2010, nearly half of those new cases were among bisexual, gay, and other (e.g., transgender) men who have sex with men. Older Black and Latino men having sex with men are at greatest risk (CDC, 2015). Although gay men represent approximately 2% of the general population, they account for nearly half of all AIDS-related deaths and new HIV infections. Regrettably, no national HIV/AIDS education programs exist for older adults, much less any specific, older LGBT population (Hillman, 2012). This is quite problematic as ageism and heterocentrism among care providers emerge as significant barriers to treatment among older LGBT adults (Fredriksen-Goldsen et al., 2014).

More than 20,000 gay men are diagnosed with prostate cancer each year, and empirical studies suggest that, like their heterosexual peers, older gay men typically maintain limited or incorrect knowledge about prostate disease, its diagnosis, and treatment (Asencio, Blank, Descartes, & Crawford, 2009). For example, older gay men may believe incorrectly that participating in rough sex increases their risk of prostate cancer, and that using a dildo instead of a penis may decrease their risk. Lower socioeconomic status is associated with less knowledge of prostate cancer, and older Black gay men appear to have the least accurate knowledge.

Many older gay, as well as older heterosexual, men also have significant concerns about how treatment for prostate cancer will affect their sexual functioning with current and future partners (Asencio et al., 2009). Although the ability to orgasm may remain intact with certain nerve sparing procedures, an inability to achieve an erection or to ejaculate may particularly challenge a gay man's sexual identity (e.g., Martinez, 2005). Other complications after treatment for prostate cancer may include urinary incontinence and rectal irritation or pain. Unfortunately, physicians often fail to discuss, with both their heterosexual and GB male patients, how various treatment options could affect their sexual functioning (Blank, 2005).

Older gay and bisexual men who engage in receptive anal sex also find themselves at increased risk for anal cancer when compared to their heterosexual peers. Linked with HPV infection, the incidence of anal cancer among gay men in the United States is higher than the incidence of cervical cancer in women. Nearly 50% of gay men with anal cancer have the HPV virus, compared to nearly 30% of heterosexual men (Daling et al., 1987). A study of HIV-negative gay men aged 18 to 89 suggests that increased age is not a protective factor; sexually active older gay men were at similar risk for developing anal cancer as younger gay men (Chin-Hong, 2005). Cigarette smoking also serves as an increased risk factor among all older men, including older gay (Daling et al., 1987) and, likely, older bisexual men.

TRANSGENDER ELDERS

Older transgender adults face significant sexual health challenges. The majority of transgender adults undergo sex reassignment surgery when they are middle-aged or older. Reasons may include waiting until retirement to avoid disclosure at work, until one's parents have died, or until enough money was saved to cover the medical expenses typically not covered by health insurance (Haber, 2009). When transgender elders broach the subject with a health care provider, they may be questioned or challenged, not about the potential risks of treatment, but about whether their transition is even "necessary" in their more advanced age (Siverskog, 2014). This blatant, ageist discrimination is consistent with some of the negative social media comments when celebrity Caitlyn Jenner announced her transition to a female identity at the age of 65.

In terms of health disparities, the Institute of Medicine (2011) reports that transgender adults typically fear discrimination from health care providers, and lack health insurance that provides coverage for sex reassignment surgery. Examples of such discrimination in health care range from providers refusing to refer to an older transgender patient by their desired gender to refusing care for postsurgical infection (Cook-Daniels & Munson, 2010). Additional disparities for transgender elders include potential increased risk for diabetes and heart disease due to long-term hormone use as well as a lack of routine and regular screenings for breast, gynecological, and prostate health care (Asencio, Blank, Descartes, & Crawford, 2009). In relation to sex reassignment surgery and hormone replacement therapy, the financial and medical risks are often greater for older transgender adults. Paying for monthly hormone treatments may be difficult on a fixed income (Cook-Daniels & Munson, 2010). Research also suggests that half of transgender elders do not have a regular health care provider, and that they may use "off-label" hormones without proper medical supervision (Williams & Freeman, 2007).

Estimates of HIV infection among MTF elders range widely from 10% to 68% (e.g., Herbst et al., 2008; Kenagy, 2005), in part because the CDC groups MTF transgender adults with men who have sex with men. Survey research suggests that more than one-third of sexually active transgender elders fail to consistently practice safe sex, and that many transgender elders (as well as all older adults in general) believe incorrectly that serial monogamy prevents the spread of STDs. Many MTF transgender elders are unaware that a surgically constructed vagina is more vulnerable to micro- and macroscopic tearing, and thus HIV infection (Kenagy & Hsieh, 2005). It also remains unclear what long-term effects may arise when HIV-positive transgender elders take both antiviral and hormone treatment therapies (Grant et al., 2010).

ISSUES IN LONG-TERM CARE

The issues surrounding sexual expression in long-term care settings are complex, particularly for older LGBT adults. Overarching themes include stigma and discrimination in which older residents, particularly those who are physically or cognitively disabled, are assumed and expected to be asexual. In contrast, surveys suggest that the majority of nursing home residents regard sex as at least "moderately important" in their lives (Aizenberg, Weizman, & Barka, 2002), and that they place significant value upon a variety of activities from kissing and hugging to masturbation and intercourse (Ginsberg, Pomerantz, & Kramer-Feeley, 2005).

The federal Nursing Home Bill of Rights (Medicare, 2007) dictates that residents have the right to dignity, privacy, and to personal belongings that do not interfere with the rights or safety of others. However, the Nursing Home Bill of Rights does not include the right to engage in LGB relationships or espouse a transgender identity per se. Even if a facility has a written policy that promotes residents' sexual rights, there is no guarantee that those residents will be able to exercise them (Parker, 2006). Much depends upon the staff, family members, and other residents. In a large-scale national study (Metlife, 2010) the majority of LG participants indicated that if placed in a nursing home, they would hide their sexual orientation out of fears of hostility and social isolation. Unfortunately, those fears may be well-founded. Qualitative analyses of ethnographic data revealed that some nursing home staff made openly negative comments about residents even suspected of being LGBT. Some transgender elders have reported that they would choose suicide rather than experience discrimination in long-term care (Cook-Daniels & Munson, 2010; Witten, 2014).

Although some long term care facilities cater specifically to LGBT residents, they represent the exception rather than the rule. (See www.gayretirementguide.com for a listing.) Concerns also exist that these LGBT-friendly communities have a long waiting list, are expensive, and are located in areas with a high cost of living (e.g., Palm Springs and San Francisco; Cahill & South, 2002). Options for low-cost LGBT-friendly retirement communities are very limited but may be expanding, as a few facilities have opened in Los Angeles and Philadelphia (Lewis, 2014).

RECOMMENDATIONS FOR BEST POLICIES AND PRACTICE

Public policy initiatives are vital to promote healthy sexuality among LGBT elders. The CDC can be encouraged to collect and provide information about specific cohorts including LGBT adults aged 50–64, 65–74, 75–84, and 85 and older as well as those who identify as bisexual and transgender. Continued funding for the Ryan White HIV/AIDS Program is essential (Cahill, Mayer, & Boswell, 2015), particularly for LGBT elders who face income disparities. The

NIH should increase its funding for LGBT-related health research. Evidence-based, national health prevention programs targeted specifically at LGBT elders, particularly in relation to HIV/AIDS, cervical, breast, and anal cancer are urgently needed. Professional health care organizations can increase the amount of training in LGBT and aging issues provided in their curriculums and require related continuing education in culturally competent care. The use of online health promotion (Bolding et al., 2004) would also be valuable.

Specific recommendations can be offered for care providers to make their practices LGBT- and aging-friendly or affirming. An essential change is to make intake and other forms LGBT inclusive. For example, questions on forms can inquire about relationship status (e.g., partnered) versus marital status and family members by choice. Intake forms should also include information about sexual health and activity, including participation in high-risk behaviors and domestic abuse, regardless of client age.

To help LGBT elders, including LGBT ethnic minority elders, feel more comfortable and accepted in a clinical setting, care providers can offer leaflets and newsletters from local and national organizations such as Services and Advocacy for GLBT Elders, and display pictures and posters featuring older LGBT families and couples from a variety of ethnic and cultural backgrounds. Care providers can also provide informational pamphlets about HIV and aging, condom use, prostate health, breast cancer, cervical cancer, anal cancer, smoking cessation, hormone therapies, substance abuse, and domestic and elder abuse. For older, potentially socially isolated rural LGBT clients, offering Internet resources can be especially important (Lee & Quam, 2013). Staff education and LGBT-friendly initiatives are especially important in long-term care. Consistent with practice guidelines from the American Geriatrics Society (2015) and the American Psychological Association (2014), care providers can engage in advocacy for individual clients as well as LGBT elders at large.

Although older LGBT adults often face significant health disparities and discrimination related to their sexuality, evidence suggests that many LGBT elders overcome these obstacles with resilience (e.g., Fredriksen-Goldsen et al., 2015) and pride. Expanded social networks including partners and close friends (e.g., family members by choice), coping and self-care strategies adopted in early life, and advocacy skills can help negate the effects of even pronounced discrimination in later life (Hash & Rogers, 2013). Care providers can be reminded to capitalize on the existing strengths of their older LGBT clients. Similarly, providing general familiarity with LGBT elders (Mabey, 2011) as well as training panels comprising older LGBT adults (Rogers, Rebbe, Gardella, Worlein, & Chamberlin, 2013), can be effective in reducing stigma and promoting education and awareness of the unique issues facing LGBT elders. Such training and continuing education can be encouraged in public policy and funding. The sexual health and authentic sexual expression of millions of LGBT elders depend upon it.

REFERENCES

Addis, S., Mavies, M., Greene, G., MacBride-Stewart, S., & Shepherd, M. (2009). The health, social care and housing needs of lesbian, gay, bisexual and transgender older people: A review of the literature. *Health and Social Care in the Community, 17*, 647–658.

Aizenberg, D., Weizman, A., & Barak, Y. (2002). Attitudes toward sexuality among nursing home residents. *Sexuality and Disability, 20*, 185–189.

American Geriatrics Society Ethics Committee. (2015). American Geriatrics Society care of lesbian, gay, bisexual, and transgender older adults position statement. *Journal of the American Geriatrics Society, 63*, 423–426.

American Psychological Association. (2014). Guidelines for psychological practice with older adults. *American Psychologist, 69*, 34–65.

Asencio, M., Blank, T., Descartes, L., & Crawford, A. (2009). The prospect of prostate cancer: A challenge for gay men's sexualities as they age. *Sexuality Research and Social Policy, 6*, 38–51.

Averett, P., Yoon, I., & Jenkins, C. L. (2012). Older lesbian sexuality: Identity, sexual behavior, and the impact of aging. *Journal of Sex Research, 49*, 495–507.

Blank, T. O. (2005). Gay men and prostate cancer: Invisible diversity. *Journal of Clinical Oncology, 23*, 2593–2596.

Bolding, G., David, M., Sherr, L., Hart, G., & Elford, J. (2004). Use of gay internet sites and views about online health promotion among men who have sex with men. *AIDS Care, 16*, 993–1001.

Cahill, S. R., Mayer, K. H., & Boswell, S. L. (2015). The Ryan White HIV/AIDS Program in the age of health care reform. *American Journal of Public Health, 105*, 1078–1085.

Cahill, S., & South, K. (2002). Policy issues affecting lesbian, gay, bisexual, and transgender people in retirement. *Generations, 26*, 49–54.

Centers for Disease Control and Prevention. (2015). *HIV among people aged 50 and older*. Retrieved from http://www.cdc.gov/hiv/group/age/olderamericans/index.html

Chin-Hong, P. V., Vitinghoff, E., Cranston, R. D., Browne, L., Buchbinder, S., Colfax, G., et al. (2005). Age-related prevalence of anal cancer precursors in homosexual men: The EXPLORE study. *Journal of the National Cancer Institute, 97*, 896–905.

Cook-Daniels, L., & Munson, M. (2010). Sexual violence, elder abuse, and sexuality of transgender adults, age 50+: Results of three surveys. *Journal of GLBT Family Studies, 6*, 142–177.

Cuypere, G. D., T'Sjoen, G., Berten, R., Selvaggi, G., Sutter, P. E., Hoebeke, P., et al. (2005). Sexual and physical health after sex reassignment surgery. *Archives of Sexual Behavior, 34*, 679–690.

Daling, J. R., Weiss, N. S., Hislop, T. G., Maden, C., Coates, R. J., Sherman, K. J., et al. (1987). Sexual practices, sexually transmitted diseases, and the incidence of anal cancer. *The New England Journal of Medicine, 317*, 973–977.

Dibble, S. L., Roberts, S. A., & Nussey, B. (2004). Comparing breast cancer risk between lesbians and their heterosexual sisters. *Women's Health Issues, 14*, 60–68.

Fassinger, R. E., & Arseneau, J. R. (2007). "I'd rather get wet than be under that umbrella": Differentiating the experiences and identities of lesbian, gay, bisexual, and transgender people. In K. J. Bieschke, R. M. Perez, & K. A. DeBord (Eds.), *Handbook of counseling and psychotherapy with lesbian, gay, bisexual, and transgender clients* (2nd ed., pp. 19–49). Washington, DC: American Psychological Association.

Fredriksen-Goldsen, K. I., Hoy-Ellis, C. P., Goldsen, J., Emlet, C. A., & Hooyman, N. R. (2014). Creating a vision for the future: Key competencies and strategies for culturally competent practice with lesbian, gay, bisexual and transgender (LGBT) older adults in the health and human services. *Journal of Gerontological Social Work, 57*, 80–107.

Fredriksen-Goldsen, K. I., Kim, H., Barkan, S. E., Muraco, A., & Hoy-Ellis, C. P. (2013). Health disparities among lesbian, gay, and bisexual older adults: Results from a population-based study. *American Journal of Public Health*, 103, 1802–1809.

Fredriksen-Goldsen, K. I., Kim, H. J., Emlet, C. A., Muraco, A., Erosheva, E. A., Hoy-Ellis, C. P., et al. (2011). *The aging and health report: Disparities and resilience among lesbian, gay, bisexual, and transgender older adults–key findings fact sheet.* Seattle, WA: Institute for Multigenerational Health.

Fredriksen-Goldsen, K. I., Kim, H., Shiu, C., Goldsen, J., & Emlet, C. A. (2015). Successful aging among LGBT older adults: Physical and mental health-related quality of life by age group. *The Gerontologist, 55*(1), 154–168.

Gelo, F. (2008). Invisible individuals: LGBT elders. *Aging Well, 1*(3), 36–40.

Ginsberg, T. B., Pomerantz, S. C., & Kramer-Feeley, V. (2005). Sexuality in older adults: Behaviours and preferences. *Age and Ageing, 34*, 475–480.

Grant, J. M., Koskovich, G., Frazer, M. S., & Bjerk, S. (2010). *Outing age 2010: Public policy issues affecting gay, lesbian, bisexual and transgender elders.* Washington, DC: National Gay and Lesbian Task Force Policy Institute.

Haber, D. (2009). Gay aging. *Gerontology and Geriatrics Education, 30*, 267–280.

Hash, K. M., & Rogers, A. (2013). Clinical practice with older LGBT clients: Overcoming lifelong stigma through strength and resilience. *Clinical Social Work Journal, 41*, 249–257.

Herbst, J. H., Jacobs, E. D., Finlayson, T. J., McKelroy, V. S., Newmann, M. S., & Crepaz, N. (2008). Estimating HIV prevalence and the risk behaviors of transgender persons in the United States. *AIDS and Behavior, 12*(1), 1–17.

Hillman, J. (2012). *Sexuality and aging: Clinical perspectives.* New York, NY: Springer Publishing.

Hughes, D., & Evans, A. (2003). Health needs of women who have sex with women. *British Medical Journal, 327*, 1739–1758.

Institute of Medicine. (2011). *The health of lesbian, gay, bisexual, and transgender people: Building a foundation for better understanding.* Washington, DC: National Academy Press.

Israel, T., & Mohr, J. J. (2004). Attitudes toward bisexual women and men: Current research, future directions. *Journal of Bisexuality, 4*, 117–134.

Kenagy, G. P. (2005). Transgender health: Findings from two needs assessment studies in Philadelphia. *Health and Social Work, 30*(1), 19–26.

Kenagy, G. P., & Hsieh, C. M. (2005). The risk less known: Female-to-male transgender persons' vulnerability to HIV infection. *AIDS Care, 17*(2), 195–207.

Lee, M. G., & Quam, J. K. (2013). Comparing supports for LGBT aging in rural versus urban areas. *Journal of Gerontological Social Work, 56*, 112–126.

Lewis, A. (2014, March 19). *The growth of gay retirement homes*. BBC News, Minneapolis. Retrieved from http://www.bbc.com/news/magazine-26554710?

Lindau, S. T., Schumm, L. P., Laumann, E. O., Levinson, W., O'Muircheataigh, C. A., & Waite, L. J. (2007). A study of sexuality and health among older adults in the United States. *The New England Journal of Medicine, 357*, 762–774.

Lovejoy, T. I., Heckman, T. G., Sikkema, K. J., Hansen, N. B., Kochman, A., Suhr, J. A., et al. (2008). Patterns and correlates of sexual activity and condom use behavior in persons 50-plus years of age living with HIV/AIDS. *AIDS and Behavior, 12*, 943–956.

Mabey, J. E. (2011). Counseling older adults in LGBT communities. *The Professional Counselor, 1*, 57–62.

Martinez, R. (2005). Prostate cancer and sex. *Journal of Gay* and *Lesbian Psychotherapy,* 9(1–2), 91–99.

McIntyre, L., Szewchuk, A., & Munro, J. (2010). Inclusion and exclusion in mid-life lesbians' experiences of the Pap test. *Culture, Health, and Sexuality, 12*, 885–898.

Medicare. (2007). *Nursing homes: Residents' rights*. Retrieved from http://www.medicare.gov/what-medicare-covers/part-a/rights-in-nursing-home.html

Metlife. (2010). Out and aging: The Metlife study of lesbian and gay baby boomers. *Journal of GLBT Family Studies, 6*, 40–57.

Parker, S. (2006). What barriers to sexual expression are experienced by older people in 24-hour care facilities. *Reviews in Clinical Gerontology, 16*, 275–270.

Rogers, A., Rebbe, R., Gardella, C., Worlein, M., & Chamberlin, M. (2013). Older LGBT adult training panels: An opportunity to educate about issues faced by the older LGBT community. *Journal of Gerontological Social Work, 56*, 580–595.

Siverskog, A. (2014). "They just don't have a clue": Transgender aging and implications for social work. *Journal of Gerontological Social Work, 57*, 2–4.

Tracy, J. K., Schluterman, N. H., & Greenberg, D. R. (2013). Understanding cervical cancer screening among lesbians: A national survey. *BioMed Central Public Health, 13*, 442–450.

Voyles, C. H. (2015). Continued disparities in lesbian, gay, and bisexual research funding at NIH. *American Journal of Public Health, 105*(Suppl. 3), e1–e2.

Waite, L. J., Laumann, E. O., Das, A., & Schumm, L. P. (2009). Sexuality: Measures of partnerships, practices, attitudes, and problems in the National Social Life, Health, and Aging Study. *The Journals of Gerontology: Series B, Psychological Sciences and Social Sciences*, 64(Suppl. 1), 56–66.

Williams, M. E., & Freeman, P. A. (2007). Transgender health: Implications for aging and caregiving. *Journal of Gay and Lesbian Social Services, 18*(3/4), 93–108.

Witten, T. M. (2014). End of life, chronic illness, and trans-identities. *Journal of Social Work in End-of-Life and Palliative Care, 10*, 34–58.

CHAPTER 3

Health and Well-Being of Transgender Elders

Tarynn M. Witten

ABSTRACT

Research on behalf of the aging lesbian, gay, bisexual, and transgender (LGBT) population has been mandated by the Institute of Medicine, the National Institutes of Health, and the Centers for Disease Control and Prevention. Despite the growing research efforts in the field of LGBT aging, focused research on the varied challenges of transgender aging remains sparse with most discussions of transgender aging included within the larger discussions of LGB aging. In this chapter, key concepts around transgender aging, health, and wellness are discussed. The reader is then provided with brief summaries of some of the transgender-related biomedical and psychosocial challenges in health care. Finally, the chapter closes with a discussion of best practices and future challenges for this growing population and for those who work on its behalf.

BACKGROUND AND KEY CONCEPTS

No matter how individuals self-identify, everyone ages, including those in the lesbian, gay, bisexual, and transgender (LGBT) population (Institute of Medicine, 2011). Aging is the global, unifying endpoint for all. And today, the first out and significant-sized cohort of transgender elders to reach either late life or end of life has finally arrived (Ippolito & Witten, 2014; Witten & Eyler, 2012).

http://dx.doi.org/10.1891/0198-8794.37.27

TERMINOLOGY

To understand aging in this population, a few key terms must be defined. It is beyond the capacity of this chapter to provide detailed descriptors that members of the global "gender nonconforming (GNC)" population use, because of the fact that they are temporal, culturally bound, often politically driven and may change with the cultural cohort and individual's evolution throughout the lifetime. For the purposes of this discussion, the word *gender* will describe the dynamics of a multidimensional variable composed of the individual's *gender self-perception* (internal identity), the individual's *gender presentation* (cultural acting; body in culture), and the interaction of that individual within a sociopolitical context. Thus, gender is an evolving process resulting from the previous constructs placed within a society at a given sociocultural-eco-political epoch. It is important to understand that gender and natal sex/birth sex have become conflated with each other, which often leads to many challenges for elders of the community (Bachman & Mussman, 2015).

While there are differences in usage across cultures and individuals, there are terms within Western cultures that are commonly used as gender descriptors. Historically, the word *transsexual* emerged as a way to describe the phenomenon of an individual who felt that he or she was born into the wrong body. Transsexual is defined here to mean individuals who chemically and/or surgically modify their bodies in an irreversible fashion to alleviate inner feelings of being out of harmony with their natal (birth) body.

The word *transgender* is a more fluid and difficult term to define. It is a historic term meant to move from the idea of trans "sexuality" to a more general and less political construct as well as to be more inclusive of individuals whose identities lay along the continuum rather than at polar ends. It is frequently interchanged with the word transsexual. For the purposes of this discussion, transgender will be understood to mean one of two things depending upon its contextual usage. First, it can be used as an umbrella term encompassing transsexuals, cross-dressers, individuals who identify as transgender, gender bending, gender blending, and a host of other terms. In a sense, transgender, as a larger group descriptor, is often conflated with the more current terms of gender nonconforming or nonbinary gender identity. The word transgender can also be used as a descriptor of an individual person's state of being. When considering individuals who are *transgender-identified*, often these persons may not see themselves as transsexual. The distinction is that transgender-identified individuals may not necessarily want to transition from their birth identity to a contra-gender identity. Rather, they only need mild or moderate transitions with such things as low doses of hormones or simply modifying their dress. This does not mean that individuals may not later decide that they really are transsexual. Rather, transgender identity indicates an intermediate state within the continuum of all possible gender states. Thus, transsexual would be a subset of transgender.

For today's trans-identified elders, the lexicon of descriptors was exceptionally restricted, namely, transgender, transsexual, and cross-dresser. It is important to understand that new linguistic topologies are emerging as younger members of the GNC population create new terms to self-describe, and they will grow older in this new philological landscape, making for a complex challenge in understanding many aspects of this younger population as it ages, including how many persons fall into these categories.

DEMOGRAPHICS

Many attempts have been made to "count" the number of trans-identified persons. The challenge lies in who is to be included or excluded. Much of the early work focused on counting transsexuals (e.g., Hoenig & Kenna, 1974). More recent work is flawed because it interchanges the term transsexual with the term transgender and reports data in terms of transgender when authors are really still counting transsexuals (Conway, 2015; Meier & Labuski, 2013). Thus, current estimates of the number of individuals who fall into the transgender, GNC, gender nonbinary population are significantly underestimated (Witten, 2003, 2015, 2016, in press). When expanding the inclusion criteria to include those who identify as transgender, GNC, and/or gender nonbinary, estimates range from as low as 1% to as high as 7% of the population (Witten & Eyler, 2012).

Estimating the numbers of transgender elders is even more elusive. The only publications solely addressing estimates of this population and including different age cohorts of transgender elders are by Witten (2003, 2014, in press). Using 1999 census data and an estimate of 1% to 3% transgender population prevalence, Witten (2003) estimated that there were approximately 347,000–1,041,000 transgender-identified persons in the United States 65+ and 4,097,020–12,291,060 individuals worldwide. Based upon more recent 2010 population estimates, Witten (in press) argues that the U.S. transgender elder population estimates should be revised to be between 1.2 million and 2.8 million trans-identified individuals 65+. There is little data available to make population estimates for GNC elder populations in non-Western countries.

CURRENT RESEARCH ON THE TRANSGENDER ELDERS

A Life Course Context of Violence, Abuse, Shame, and Invisibility

Research has demonstrated that a large proportion of today's trans-identified individuals have grown up within a psychosocial context of violence

(Fredriksen-Goldsen et al., 2014), biomedical/psychosocial abuse (Kattari & Hasche, 2015; Willging, Salvador, & Kano, 2006a, 2006b), and invisibility (Witten & Carpenter, 2015). Persons who identify as "gender variant" (Witten & Eyler, 2012) are frequently subjected to discrimination, sexual violence, and elder abuse (Cook-Daniels & Munson, 2008). For example, surveys of transgender adults aged 50+ found that more than one-third of the respondents had experienced discrimination in health care (Aghajanian, 2015) and continue to do so. Moreover, given that many of the current elders of the trans-population grew up in this adverse environment, they are fearful and/or unwilling to interact with health care providers (Rachlin, Green, & Lombardi, 2008). As a result, many trans-identified individuals do not make use of medical care facilities even if they have insurance. For example, many have not had a physical or been to the dentist in years and only seek care as a matter of last resort.

It is now well-documented that early and life-course adversity, violence, and abuse has an effect on lifelong health (Firth 2014; Moffitt & Klaus-Grawe, 2013) including mortality (Felitti et al., 1998), active life expectancy (Montez & Hayward, 2014), morbidity (Shalev et al., 2013), mental health (Agahi, Shaw, Benjamin, & Fors, 2014), and biomedical health in mid-to-later life (Kreatsoulas, Hassan, Subramanian, & Fleegler, 2015). Fredriksen-Goldsen, Kim, Shiu, Goldsen, and Emlet (2015) found that,

> the [their] transgender older adult participants had significantly poorer health in terms of physical health, disability, depressive symptomatology, and perceived more stress than the non-transgender LGB older adult participants, controlling for key background characteristics. These findings suggest that the patterns of adverse health identified among transgender adults in early and middle adulthood persist into later life. (p. 155)

Given what is now known about how early life factors can affect later-life psychosocial and biomedical health (Witten, 2004, 2008), it is natural to ask how life-course events can modulate a trans-identified individual's later-life needs, challenges, frailties, resilience, and preparations. Currently, there is limited research on how transgender-identified older adults are aging. Fredriksen-Goldsen, Kim, and Goldsen (2014), in one of the first national surveys of LGBT older adults, reported that transgender older adults have lower levels of self-acceptance than LGB or heterosexual older adults. Moreover, social stigma often leads to social isolation, as more than half of transgender adults aged 55+ reported losing close friends and 40% losing contact with children due to their gender identity (Grant et al., 2011), and almost half of these older adults (44%) live alone (Fredriksen-Goldsen et al., 2014) compared to 18% of the general population (MetLife Mature Market Institute, 2010). It is within this psychosocial context that today's trans aging cohort has evolved to their elder status and must navigate later-life and end-of-life challenges.

Biomedical Aspects of Transgender Aging

Very few articles have focused on the biomedical care of transgender-identified elders (Fabbre, 2015; Witten & Eyler, 2012, 2016). Until additional, carefully executed research on the care of transgender older adults is conducted, health care providers must typically draw conclusions from evidence-based research regarding care of nontransgender (cisgender) geriatric patients. However, certain things can be said about a number of important trans-related, biomedical care issues.

Smoking and Substance Use

Substance abuse in the general elder population is a well-known problem. Addiction is higher in older adults who smoke, drink, or suffer from depression. Poverty, dementia, bereavement, caring for an ill partner, negative social stereotypes, and poor physical health place older adults at high risk of substance abuse and addiction. Current estimates of alcohol abuse in the older population range from 3.7% to as much as 10%. Drug abuse, specifically related to prescription drugs, is estimated at as much as 10% among individuals aged 50+. Substance abuse among those 60+ (including misuse of prescription drugs) currently affects about 17% of this population. By 2020, the number of older adults with substance abuse problems is expected to double (Ippolito & Witten, 2014).

It is not clear whether LGBT people are more likely than non-LGBTs to use alcohol and drugs, have a higher rate of substance abuse, are less likely to abstain from use, and are more likely to drink heavily in later life. It is known that, in the LGB population, heterosexism and homophobia are often related to increased substance abuse; there is no reason to assume otherwise for the transgender-identified population. However, little is currently known about substance abuse in the elder transgender-identified population (Witten & Eyler, 2016).

New studies suggest that for transgender and GNC persons, suicidality, substance abuse, and tobacco use are further exacerbated. Suggested reasons are homelessness, ongoing microaggressions, loss of employment, social anxiety, diminished or lost social support network (Erosheva, Kim, Emlet, & Fredriksen-Goldsen, 2015), and internalized transphobia. The ongoing abuse, violence, and isolation due to gender identity challenges can create additional struggles for individuals. High rates of smoking have been documented in the transgender-identified population with prior studies indicating two times the smoking rate among LGBT-identified persons compared to the overall U.S. population (Fredriksen-Goldsen, Kim, Barkan, Muraco, & Hoy-Ellis, 2013).

Hormones in Older Adulthood

Treatment with hormonal medications is a medically necessary therapy for many persons with gender dysphoria, or an incongruence between one's experience/expressed gender and assigned gender (Coleman et al., 2012). Best clinical practice guidelines for use of estrogens and androgens by transgender older adults are considerably less well defined. The aging process affects the effectiveness of contra-gender hormones. While much is known about overall pharmacologic and hormonal changes of aging (Shi, 2011), research involving transgender older persons using supplemental hormones is much less robust, and prescribing practices often must be extrapolated from data regarding nontransgender populations. For example, the risks of estrogen use among nontranssexual women increase with age, and it is very likely that transgender women are similarly affected. Many transgender older adults are willing to accept the risks that accompany treatment with estrogens or androgens to gain the psychological benefits that congruence between the psychological gender and the physical body can provide. No clinical data is available regarding the biomedical experience of older trans women. It follows that estrogen use in this population must be considered based upon the data around the biomedical, postmenopausal estrogen supplementation among nontransgender women. Data on mortality and morbidity associated with androgen use suggests that its use in transgender males is generally safe (Asscheman et al., 2011). However, there is marginal long-term data concerning testosterone use by older trans men.

HIV in Later Life

Concern around HIV/AIDS in the transgender population has been escalating (Hoffman, 2015). Nevertheless, little is known about HIV/AIDs in the current cohort of trans elders (Witten, 2004). Moreover, little is known about the intersectionality of race (Nemoto, Operario, Keatley, & Villegas, 2004) with trans-status and aging. Older adults may be particularly at risk for exposure to HIV and other sexually transmittable infections due to having come of age in an era during which HIV and other sexual disease infections were not of concern. Furthermore, many transgender older persons report not having used any safer sex techniques during first dating experiences in the new gender presentation, as they are not familiar with or have not yet understood the reasons for such protection. In addition, younger generations of trans-identified persons with HIV/AIDS may be living longer due to better medical treatment.

Psychosocial Aspects of Transgender Aging

Intimacy and Sexuality

Health care perspectives concerning elder intimacy and sexuality are not typically encouraging. Most eldercare facilities do not have the means to support sexual behaviors of elder clients. Often, such acts are not viewed to be in the lexicon of older individuals' needs. When the physical corpus does not reflect the gender presentation, as in individuals who are living in one gender identity but have not undergone genital surgery, sexuality and intimacy can create extreme difficulties for both the elder and the care staff.

Spirituality, Faith, and Religiosity

Literature has established the importance of spirituality, faith, and religiosity for the general geriatric population on overall positive aging and dealing with end-of-life challenges. More recently, research has addressed the role and importance of spirituality, faith, and religiosity in the transgender-identified population (Hopwood & Witten, in press; Tabaac & Witten, 2016). Despite this importance, individuals who are transgender-identified often face exclusion, penalties, or other deleterious behaviors on the part of spiritual organizations due to beliefs that being transgender-identified is a sin (Kidd & Witten, 2007).

Depression, Anxiety, and Suicidality

Anxiety and depression are common among the general aging population. While there are no specific estimates on anxiety and depression prevalence in the general elder transgender and GNC population, it is easy to hypothesize that levels of anxiety and depression are high, given their overall history and ongoing experience of violence and abuse. General studies of the trans-identified population show that levels of depression and anxiety are far above those in the nontransgender population. Budge, Adelson, and Howard (2013) find that the rates of depression (51.4% for transgender women; 48.3% for transgender men) and anxiety (40.4% for transgender women; 47.5% for transgender men) far surpass the rates of those for the general population. Bockting, Miner, Romine, Hamilton, and Coleman (2013) find a high prevalence of clinical depression (44.1% overall), anxiety (33.2% overall), and somatization challenges (27.5% overall). They found that peer support moderated the relationship between these disorders and minority stress. Other studies find similar results (Nuttbrock et al., 2014a, 2014b) though only Fredriksen-Goldsen et al. (2014) discuss the mental health status of transgender older adults, finding significantly elevated levels of anxiety and depression with respect to the general population.

In addition, depression around lost time in the target identity, particularly among older male-to-female transsexuals, can create challenges leading to abuse of substances. Increased medical health challenges delaying desired transitions or possibly stopping them, confounding effects of disability, HIV/AIDS, hepatitis C, prior silicone injections, and mental health factors can all lead to depression, social isolation, and poverty, all of which have been shown to have long-term effects on later-life mortality and morbidity (Fredriksen-Goldsen et al., 2014).

The American Association of Marriage and Family Therapy (n.d.) reports that in 2002 the annual suicide rate for persons 65+ was 15/100,000 with the rate going to 17/100,000 in the 75–84-year-old age group. Moreover, in 2013, overall U.S. 65+ years old suicide rate was 16/100,000 (Krans, 2015) while the U.S. 65+ suicide rates per state ranged from 7.7/100,000 to as high as 30.5/100,000 (American Association of Suicidology, 2015). The 85+ suicide rate was 18.6/100,000 (Krans, 2015). However, it is also thought that elder suicide may be underreported by as much as 40%.

The literature on trans-suicides is growing (Haas et al., 2011), with estimates as high as 80% for those who have thought of suicide and 50% or more who have attempted it. There is little data on suicidality in the elder trans-identified population. Nevertheless, it is no surprise that a number of the respondents to the TransMetLife Survey (TMLS) had euthanasia as part of a life plan because they feared later-life mistreatment or dementia (Witten, 2014). The idea of living in long-term care is one filled with the fear of being abused, having one's person violated, receiving incomplete or inaccurate care, or worse. As a result, many trans-persons have plans to go back into the closet (reverse surgeries where possible) or commit suicide if they need to relocate and receive care in a long-term care facility.

Late and End-of-life Concerns

The TMLS examined the later- and end-of-life preparation and concerns of the global transgender-identified population (Witten, 2014, 2015, 2016, in press). Respondents were asked to rank-order a list of concerns about aging. The top four concerns were: becoming unable to care for myself; becoming sick or disabled; becoming dependent upon others; and becoming confused or demented.

Areas of greatest concern were around being able to function independently because of a lack of supports or because of financial inability to afford care. The cumulative legacy of financial discrimination faced by many trans-identified persons who, once they transitioned, were more likely to have periods of unemployment and/or working in low-wage jobs manifests itself in fears of being unable to afford care that they needed to remain independent. Further, privacy deteriorates with elevated physical dependency, particularly with respect to bathroom-related functions such as toileting and bathing. Trans-identified individuals whose gender self-perception and gender presentation are not matched with their physical corpus may be particularly fearful of abuse on the part of end-of-life health care workers (Witten, 2014). Pain management at end of life is also a concern, and many trans-persons require palliative care. However, there is no focused research on end-of-life palliative care for trans elders. What little is mentioned occurs within the context of end-of-life issues for the LGBT population (Rawlings, 2012).

Witten (2014) has shown that elders of the current trans elder cohort are ill-prepared for other later-life and end-of-life challenges. While many of the male-to-female respondents had wills, very few female-to-male and other trans-identifications did, and a large number of all trans-identities had no advanced directives, documents on disposition of the body, or powers of attorney, for example. Few had directives around memorials, legacy, or funereal arrangements.

Many trans-persons fear that in their last days they will be disrespected and their last wishes will not be carried out (Witten, 2014, 2015, 2016, in press). They speak of the importance of being able to die with grace and in their true identities. It is important that advance planning take place to respect the needs of all concerned in the end-of-life course of the trans-person. Trans-persons have spoken of being denied funereal ceremony rights, burial rights in the church graveyard, marriage ceremonies, last rights, and even access to spiritual counseling when needed because they were transgender-identified. More recently, a transgender-identified woman died and was presented as a man in her casket (Rothaus, 2014). For individuals and families of transgender-identified individuals, denial of access to spiritual care and end-of-life rights is a significant loss. It is important to realize that these challenges also impact the family, friends, and allies of the trans-person.

Concluding Trends and Future Directions for the Aging Trans-Population

Throughout this discussion, the lack of research on various aspects of the biomedical and psychosocial aspects of transgender aging has been noted. Moreover, there will be new cohorts that have different life experiences, and they will also be getting older. Young trans-persons must be educated around long-term fiscal planning in all aspects of their lives. Even at young ages, individuals should have legal documents in place that will advocate for them in case they cannot speak for themselves. Nothing is known about their perceptions, preparations, or experiences of the aging process. Further, within all of these cohorts, next to nothing is known about how intersectionalities such as race, socioeconomic status, gender self-perception, and self-expression and sexual identity play a part in the lived experience of growing older. Similarly, nothing about trans aging within the street sex-worker, the military, or the prison system is known.

The aging of the "baby-boomer" generation carries with it the significant likelihood that health care practitioners in all areas will see trans-identified individuals within their practices. Documented ongoing marginalization of the elder trans-population diminishes the likelihood of their receiving needed care in later- and end-of-life situations. Education at all levels is important (Nemoto, Sausa, Operario, & Keatley, 2006). Students in health care and other disciplines need to learn about the needs of both current and upcoming generations of trans-persons and their caregivers. For example, medical schools need to make educational opportunities available for students to learn about treating trans-identified clients. Nursing, dental, and social work programs likewise need programs relevant to their students to teach them how to care for trans-persons entering their respective care facilities.

Mental health practitioners need to focus on interventions that reduce avoidant coping strategies, address body-centered issues, increase social support network connections and peer support systems, develop health promoting physical and mental activities, incorporate spirituality, faith, and religiosity where appropriate and focus on person-centered care. The psychologist/psychiatrist/social worker should understand that many factors mediate mental health. Among these are age, employment, transition status (early, late, never), history of violence and abuse, and current social support. Further, resiliency among those in this population needs to be considered. For example, in the face of the endemic history of violence, abuse, and invisibility for trans-persons, when asked if they had aged positively, a significant number of them indicated they had (van Wagenen, Driskell, & Bradford, 2013; Witten, 2013).

Greater effort needs to be made to reach out into the world itself to educate non-trans-persons about the challenges around being so identified. There is still a significant lack of understanding, misinformation, and confusion around what a transgender identity is about. This creates fear, which can lead to violence and abuse.

CONCLUSIONS

> ". . . No one ever chooses to be transgendered and punished for it by being cut off from what society has to offer"
>
> TMLS respondent (Witten, in press)

Aging is a complex process. It involves an interaction of biomedical, psychosocial, institutional, organizational, economic, and political factors. Within this complex reality, transgender-identified and gender-queer-identified persons must face the inevitable and inexorable processes of aging. They must do so in the face of varying degrees of past, present, and future stigma, abuse, violence, marginalization, invisibility, erasure, ignorance, and multiple other disenfranchisements that can and often do make their lives difficult to navigate. They face economic disparities, educational inequalities, and ongoing barriers to access needed health care at all levels of the health care organizational hierarchy. They also risk disclosure through medical records, as medical and social service histories and intakes, in determining their needs, can make them vulnerable to numerous injustices as they are forced to identify their transgendered nature. This "outing" can place them in a situation of being isolated from their families, reducing their income and future financial capacity, reducing their social network system, denying them access to their spiritual/faith/religious support system, and making them invisible. The risk of later-life and end-of-life abuse, violence, maltreatment, and denial of care in retirement and nursing home facilities has created a generation of trans-persons who talk of reversing their transitions, going back into the closet, and even committing suicide before entering such facilities.

The process of successful aging, achievement of gerotranscendence and subsequent graceful exits, like retirement, must be planned and carefully monitored for positive accomplishment. And those who work with elders of this population are cautioned to be sensitive to these factors and to act in an understanding and compassionate fashion.

REFERENCES

Agahi, N., Shaw, B. A., Benjamin, A., & Fors, A. (2014). Social and economic conditions in childhood and the progression of functional health problems from midlife into old age. *Journal of Epidemiology and Community Health*, *68*(8), 734–740.

Aghajanian, L. (2015). *Aging trans people are systematically locked out of the healthcare system*. Retrieved from http://www.newsweek.com/2015/11/13/trans-people-cant-get-health-care-390375.html

American Association for Marriage and Family Therapy. (n.d.). *Suicide in the elderly*. Retrieved from http://www.aamft.org/iMIS15/AAMFT/Content/Consumer_Updates/Suicide_in_the_Elderly.aspx

American Association of Suicidology. (2015). *Suicide in the United States 2012*. Retrieved from http://www.suicidology.org/Portals/14/docs/Resources/FactSheets/USA2012.pdf

Asscheman, H., Giltay, E. J., Megens, J. A. J., de Ronde, W., van Trotsenburg, M. A. A., & Gooren, L. J. G. (2011). A long-term follow-up study of mortality in transsexuals receiving treatment with cross-sex hormones. *European Journal of Endocrinology, 164*(4), 635–642.

Bachman, G. A., & Mussman, B. (2015). The aging population: imperative to uncouple sex and gender to establish "gender equal" health care. *Maturitas*, *80*(4), 421–425.

Bockting, W. O., Miner, M. H., Romine, R. E. S., Hamilton, A., & Coleman, E. (2013). Stigma, mental health, and resilience in an online sample of the U.S. transgender population. *American Journal of Public Health, 103*(5), 943–951.

Budge, S. L., Adelson, J. L., & Howard, K. A. S. (2013). Anxiety and depression in transgender individuals: The roles of transition status, loss, social support and coping. *Journal of Consulting and Clinical Psychology*, *81*(3), 545–557.

Coleman, E., Bockting, W., Botzer, M., Cohen-Kettenis, P., DeCuypere, G., Feldman, J. et al. (2012). Standards of care for the health of transsexual, transgender and gender nonconforming people, Version 7. *International Journal of Transgenderism*, *12*(4), 165–232.

Conway, L. (2015). *How many of us are there?* Retrieved from http://ai.eecs.umich.edu/people/conway/TS/TSprevalence.html

Cook-Daniels, L., & Munson, M. (2008). *Sexual violence, elder abuse, and sexuality of transgender adults age 50+: Results of three surveys.* Retrieved from www.forge-forward.org/docs/APA2008_trans_elders_3surveys.pdf

Erosheva, E. A., Kim, H. J., Emlet, C., & Fredricksen-Goldsen, K. I. (2015). Social networks of lesbian, gay, bisexual and transgender older adults. *Research on Aging*, *38*(1), 98–123.

Fabbre, V. D. (2015). Gender transitions in later life: A queer perspective on successful aging. *The Gerontologist*, *55*(1), 144–153.

Felitti, V. J., Anda, R. F., Nordenberg, D., Williamson, D. F., Spitz, A. M., Edwards, V., et al. (1998). Relationship of childhood abuse and household dysfunction to many of the leading causes of death in adults. *American. Journal of Preventive Medicine*, *14*(4), 245–258.

Firth, M. T. (2014). Childhood abuse and depressive vulnerability in clients with gender dysphoria. *Counseling and Psychotherapy Research*, *14*(4), 297–305.

Fredriksen-Goldsen, K. I., Cook-Daniels, L., Kim, H. J., Erosheva, E. A., Emlet, C. A., Hoy-Ellis, C. P., et al. (2014). Physical and mental health of transgender older adults: An at-risk and underserved population. *The Gerontologist*, *54*(3), 488–500.

Fredriksen-Goldsen, K. I., Kim, H.-J., Barkan, S. E., Muraco, A., & Hoy-Ellis, C. P. (2013). Health disparities among lesbian, gay, and bisexual older adults: Results from a population-based study. *American Journal of Public Health*, *103*(10), 1802–1809.

Fredriksen-Goldsen, K. I., Kim, H.-J., Shiu, C., Goldsen, J., & Emlet, A. C. (2015). Successful aging among LGBT older adults: Physical and mental health-related quality of life by age group. *The Gerontologist*, *55*(1), 154–168.

Grant, J., Mottet, M., Tanis, J., Harrison, J., Keisling, H., & Keisling, M. (2011). *Injustice at every turn: A report of the national transgender discrimination survey*. Washington: National Center for Transgender Equality and National Gay and Lesbian Task Force. Retrieved from http://endtransdiscrimination.org/report.html

Haas, A. P., Eliason, M., Mays, V. M., Mathy, R. M., Cochran, A. D., D'Augelli, A. R., et al. (2011). Suicide and suicide risk in lesbian, gay, bisexual and transgender populations: Review and recommendations. *Journal of Homosexuality*, *58*(1), 10–51.

Hoenig, J., & Kenna, C. (1974). The prevalence of transsexualism in England and Wales. *British Journal of Psychiatry*, *124*(579), 181–190.

Hoffman, B. R. (2015). The interaction of drug use, sex work and HIV among transgender women. *Substance Use and Misuse*, *49*(8), 1049–1053.

Hopwood, R., & Witten, T. M. (in press). Religion and spirituality. In A. Singh and L. M. Dickey (Eds.), *American Psychological Association guidelines on psychological practice with transgender and gender non-conforming clients.* Washington, DC: American Psychological Association.

Institute of Medicine. (2011). *The health of lesbian, gay, bisexual and transgender people: Building a foundation for better understanding*. Washington, DC: The National Academies Press.

Ippolito, J., & Witten, T. M. (2014). Aging. In L. Erickson-Schroth (Ed.), *Trans bodies, trans selves* (pp. 476–500). New York, NY: Oxford University Press.

Kattari, S. K., & Hasche. (2015). Differences across age groups in transgender and gender non-conforming people's experiences of health care discrimination, harassment and victimization. *Journal of Aging and Health*, *28*(2), 285–306.

Kidd, J. D., & Witten, T. M. (2007). Assessing spirituality, religiosity and faith in the transgender community: A case study in violence and abuse – implications for the aging transgender community and for Gerontological Research. *Journal of Religious Gerontology*, *20*(1–2), 29–62.

Krans, B. (2015). *Baby boomer suicide rate rising, may go higher with age*. Retrieved from http://www.healthline.com/health-news/baby-boomer-suicide-rate-rising-031515#1

Kreatsoulas, C., Hassan, A., Subramanian, S. V., & Fleegler, E. W. (2015). Social disparities among youth and the impact on their health. *Adolescent Health, Medicine and Therapeutics, 2015*(6), 37–45.

Meier, S. C., & Labuski, C. M. (2013). The demographics of the transgender population. In A. K. Baumle (Ed.), *International handbooks of population* (Vol. 5, pp. 289–327). New York, NY: Springer Publishing.

MetLife Mature Market Institute. (2010). *Still out still aging: The MetLife study of lesbian and gay baby boomers*. Retrieved from http://www.metlife.com/assets/cao/mmi/publications/studies/2010/mmi-still-out-still-aging.pdf

Moffitt, T. E., & Klaus-Grawe 2012 Think Tank. (2013). Childhood exposure to violence and lifelong health: Clinical intervention science and stress biology research join forces. *Developmental Psychopathology*, *25*(4 Pt. 2), 1619–1634.

Montez, J. K., & Hayward, M. D. (2014). Cumulative childhood adversity, educational attainment and active life expectancy. *Demography*, *51*(2), 413–435.

Nemoto, T., Operario, D., Keatley, J., & Villegas, D. (2004). Social context of HIV risk behaviours among male-to-female transgenders of colour. *AIDS Care*, *16*(6), 724–735.

Nemoto, T., Sausa, L. A., Operario, D., & Keatley, J. (2006). Need for HIV/AIDS education and intervention for MTF transgenders. *Journal of Homosexuality*, *51*(1), 183–201.

Nuttbrock, L., Bockting, W., Rosenblum, A., Hwahng, S., Mason, M., Macri, M., et al. (2014a). Gender abuse, depressive symptoms and HIV and other sexually transmitted infections among male-to-female transgender persons: A three-year prospective study. *American Journal of Public Health*, *103*(2), 300–307.

Nuttbrock, L., Bockting, W., Rosenblum, A., Hwahng, S., Mason, M., Macri, M., et al. (2014b). Gender abuse and major depression among transgender women: A prospective study of vulnerability and resilience. *American Journal of Public Health, 104*(11), 2191–2198.

Rachlin, K., Green, J., & Lombardi, E. (2008). Utilization of health care among female-to-male transgender individuals in the United States. *Journal of Homosexuality, 54*(3), 243–258.

Rawlings, D. (2012). End-of-life care considerations for gay, lesbian, bisexual and transgender individuals. *International Journal of Palliative Nursing, 18*(1), 29–34.

Rothaus, S. (2014). *Transgender woman dies suddenly, presented at funeral in open casket as a man.* Retrieved from http://www.miamiherald.com/news/local/community/gay-south-florida/article4055600.html#/tabPane=tabs-30a8a142-17

Shalev, I., Moffitt, T. E., Sugden, K., Williams, B., Houts, R. M., Danese, A., et al. (2013). Exposure to violence during childhood is associated with telomere erosion from 5 to 10 years of age: A longitudinal study. *Molecular Psychiatry, 18*(5), 576–581.

Shi, S., & Klotz, U. (2011). Age-related changes in pharmacokinetics. *Current Drug Metabolism, 12*(7), 1389–2002.

Tabaac, A., & Witten, T. M. (2016). Trans* people and religion/spirituality. In A. E. Goldberg (Ed.), *The SAGE Encyclopedia of LGBTQ Studies.* New York, NY: Sage Publications.

van Wagenen, A., Driskell, J., & Bradford, J. (2013). "I'm still raring to go": Successful aging among lesbian, gay, bisexual and transgender older adults. *Journal of Aging Studies, 27*(1), 1–14.

Willging, C. E., Salvador, M., & Kano, M. (2006a). Unequal treatment: Mental health care for sexual and gender minority groups in a rural state. *Psychiatric Services, 57*(6), 867–870.

Willging, C. E., Salvador, M., & Kano, M. (2006b). Pragmatic help seeking: How sexual and gender minority groups access mental health care in a rural state. *Psychiatric Services, 57*(6), 871–874.

Witten, T. M. (in press). When my past returns: Loss of self and personhood–dementia and the trans-person. In S. Westwood & E. Price (Eds.), *Lesbian, gay, bisexual and trans* individuals living with Dementia: Theoretical, practical and rights-based perspectives.* New York, NY: Routledge Press.

Witten, T. M. (2003). Transgender aging: An emerging population and an emerging need. *Review Sexologies, XII*(4), 15–20.

Witten, T. M. (2004). Life course analysis: The courage to search for something more; Middle adulthood issues in the transgender and intersex community. *Journal of Human Behavior in the Social Environment, 8*(3/4), 189–224.

Witten, T. M. (2008). Transgender bodies, identities, and healthcare: Effects of perceived and actual violence and abuse. In J. J. Kronenfeld (Ed.), *Research in the sociology of healthcare: Inequalities and disparities in health care and health – Concerns of patients. v. 25* (pp. 225–249). Oxford, England: Elsevier JAI.

Witten, T. M. (2013). It's not all darkness: Resilience, robustness and successful aging in the trans-community. *LGBT Health*, *1*(1), 24–33.

Witten, T. M. (2014). End of life, chronic illness and trans-identities. *Journal of Social Work in End-of-Life and Palliative Care*, *10*, 1–26.

Witten, T. M. (2015). Elder transgender lesbians: Exploring the intersection of aging, lesbian sexual identity and transgender identity. *Journal of Lesbian Studies*, *19*, 1–17.

Witten, T. M. (2016). Elder transgender bisexuals: Exploring the intersection of aging, bisexual sexual identity and transgender identity. *Journal of Bisexual Studies, 16*(1), 58–80.

Witten, T. M. (in press). To boldly go where few trans have gone before: Facing the intersectional challenges of aging and of being a gender non-conforming identities adult. *Generations*.

Witten, T. M., & Carpenter, B. (2015). *Invisibility squared: The challenges of living as a transgender older adult*. Retrieved from http://psychologybenefits.org/2015/03/09/invisibility-squared-the-challenges-of-living-as-a-transgender-older-adult

Witten, T. M., & Eyler, A. E. (2016). Care of aging transgender and gender non-conforming individuals. In R. Ettner, S. Monstrey, & A. E. Eyler (Eds.), *Principles of transgender medicine and surgery* (2nd ed., pp. 344–378). Binghamton, NY: Haworth Press.

Witten, T. M., & Eyler, A. E. (Eds.). (2012). *Lesbian, gay, bisexual, and transgender aging: Challenges in research, practice, and policy*. Baltimore, MD: Johns Hopkins University Press.

CHAPTER 4

Stigma and Special Issues for Bisexual Older Adults

Kristin S. Scherrer

ABSTRACT

Though there have been considerable inroads in scholarly knowledge about gay, lesbian, and to a lesser extent, transgender, older adults, considerably less is known about bisexual older adults. Scholarship that focuses on bisexual older adults indicates that they experience unique challenges based on the intersections of their age and sexual orientation. This chapter provides an overview of extant literature on older bisexual adults, utilizing the lens of intersectionality to further theorize about how other identities (e.g., race, gender, class) shape the experiences of older bisexual people. Central to this analysis is the role that biphobia, or the negative attitudes and stereotypes about bisexuality, plays in the lives of older bisexual people. Best practices for helping professionals working with this population are reviewed.

INTRODUCTION

Considerable inroads have been made in recent years in extending knowledge about the experiences of gay and lesbian older adults and to a more limited extent, bisexual and transgender older adults. Scholarship indicates that gay, lesbian, bisexual, and transgender (GLBT) older adults face considerable challenges in

http://dx.doi.org/10.1891/0198-8794.37.43

many realms of life. For example, recent scholarship has illuminated the inequalities and challenges that older GLBT people contend with in regard to physical and sexual health, substance abuse, coping with grief and loss, legal issues, family support, and community and social services (Kimmel, Rose, & David, 2006; Orel & Fruhauf, 2014; Witten & Eyler, 2012). Despite these important advances in knowledge about the roles that sexual orientation and gender identity play in older people's lives, comparably less is known about the experiences of older adults who identify as bisexual.

Focusing on the experiences of bisexual older adults is important for several reasons. First, bisexual people face unique challenges relative to their identity, as *biphobia* (Israel & Mohr, 2004; Ochs, 1996; Rodriguez-Rust, 2002), or the negative attitudes toward and stereotypes about bisexual people, is pervasive (Herek, 2002; Spalding & Peplau, 1997). As is discussed later, biphobia can have profound implications for bisexual older adults' health and well-being. Second, bisexual people are the demographic majority among gay, lesbian and bisexual (GLB) identities (Egan, Edelman, & Sherrill, 2007; Hebenick et al., 2010; Mosher, Chandra, & Jones, 2005). It is therefore imperative that service providers who work with older adults understand the unique issues that bisexual individuals face, above and beyond the general issues that are shared by the GLBT community more broadly. Third, research shows that bisexual people exhibit more challenges regarding mental health issues when compared to lesbian, gay, and heterosexual individuals (Bertsch, 2014; Dodge & Sandfort, 2007; Jorm, Korten, Rodgers, Jacomb, & Christensen, 2002; Kertzner, Meyer, Frost, & Stirratt, 2009), indicating that this is an identity group that could benefit from additional support from culturally competent health and mental health practitioners. Last, most of the extant knowledge about bisexual older adults is based on research that combines the experiences of GLB older adults (Keppel & Firestein, 2007). As Keppel and Firestein (2007) note in their review of research on bisexual older adults,

> It is startling to realize how little attention is being directed toward older bisexual men and women by organizations focused on LGBT aging that nominally include *bisexuals* in the titles of their organizations and in their mission statements. (p. 168)

Although there are many shared experiences among GLB people, there is still a relative lack of knowledge about older bisexual people specifically.

Before continuing, it will be useful to briefly review a few additional concepts that are central to this analysis. In this chapter, the term *bisexual* can be understood as an identity adopted by a person often meant to convey attraction to individuals of more than one gender category. While this definition may offer some clarity as to how this term will be used in this chapter, it is by no means a universally shared definition, nor should it be expected that this definition would resonate with all people who identify as bisexual. Indeed, as Rodriguez-Rust (2012) reminds us, there is great diversity among those who identify as bisexual, and one such element of this diversity is in the meaning of the concept bisexuality. A concept that is closely related to biphobia is that of *monosexism*, or the assumption that individuals will be attracted to people of only one gender (Bradford, 2004; Rodriguez-Rust, 2002). A final important concept is that of *intersectionality*. This chapter utilizes the theoretical lens of intersectionality to better understand how other salient identities, such as race, age, or gender, reciprocally shape bisexual older adults' experiences. The concept of intersectionality acknowledges that one's social identities are inextricably interconnected and that one must attend to differences within identity categories when seeking understanding about identity-based experiences (Bowleg, 2012; Collins, 2000). Intersectional understandings of identities enable more complex and nuanced understandings of people's lived experiences, for instance in being able to understand how the experience of being bisexual is shaped by other social identities such as gender, race, or age. In this analysis, the concept of intersectionality is employed to examine how bisexual older adults' experiences are shaped by other identities (e.g., race, gender, age) as well as for theorizing about how these multiple identities shape the needs of this community.

This chapter addresses the gap in knowledge about bisexual older adults. As Cohler (2005) indicates, "there has been very little study of men and women who self-define as bisexual in a continuing preference across the course of life" (p. 87). This chapter first provides an overview of the challenges that are experienced by bisexual older adults. Scholarly literature indicates that bisexual individuals contend with biphobic stereotypes, although the ways that biphobia plays out for older adults may differ from their younger counterparts. It then examines existing literature on best practices for serving this population. Specifically, this chapter provides a review of how social service providers may intervene with older bisexual people in more culturally competent ways.

CHALLENGES FOR BISEXUAL OLDER ADULTS

The pervasive, negative attitudes about and stereotypes of bisexual people represent a significant challenge for bisexual older adults. One stereotype about bisexuality is that it is perceived as a temporary or otherwise inauthentic identity. Monosexist beliefs undergird these biphobic attitudes in positing that attraction to people of more than one gender is immature or that this identity is transitory. Furthermore, this stereotype is gendered. Men are more frequently understood by others as *really* gay, and women are more frequently understood as *really* heterosexual (Barker, Bowes-Catton, Iantaffi, Cassidy, & Brewer, 2008; Eliason, 2001; Esterberg, 2006; Horowitz & Newcomb, 1999; Scherrer, Kazyak, & Schmitz, 2015). In other words, the expectations of these monosexist beliefs have very different outcomes depending on the gender of the bisexual person. As with gender, age is also important for how this particular stereotype may be interpreted by others. Although research has not examined this empirically, it may be that this stereotype is particularly salient for younger bisexual people who are chronologically closer to a developmental time period marked by self-discovery and change. In contrast, bisexual older adults, who by virtue of their age may be less likely to be seen as early in their identity development process, may be less likely to be seen as developmentally immature. Ironically, the age status of bisexual older adults may protect them from stereotypes about their identity as immature or transitory. Taken together, these examples illustrate how important it is to examine sexual orientation using an intersectional lens, to better appreciate variations within this group.

Another common stereotype about bisexual people pertains to the strong sexual drive of bisexual people, and a conception that bisexual people will have sex with "anything that moves" (Ochs, 1996). Furthermore, bisexual people may be seen as not interested in, or capable of, monogamous relationships. Another component of this stereotype is the belief that bisexual people are carriers of sexually transmitted infections (Eliason, 2001; Mohr et al., 2009), or that bisexual people are untrustworthy or unreliable partners (Eliason, 2001; Spalding & Peplau, 1997). These stereotypes may be heightened for bisexual men (Goetstouwers, 2006; Israel & Mohr, 2004; Spalding & Peplau, 1997; Worth, 2003) and even more so for bisexual men of color (Henderson, 2009; Malebranche, Arriola, Jenkins, Dauria, & Patel, 2010) further illustrating the intersectional nature of these stereotypes when considering gender and race. When examining bisexual and age-related identities intersectionally, it may be that some stereotypes about bisexual people as hypersexual may be inhibited for older adults, given dissonant stereotypes of older adults as less interested in sex or as asexual (Hodson & Skeen, 1994; Scherrer, 2009).

These stereotypes have a number of implications for bisexual older people. One way that biphobic stereotypes may emerge for older bisexual people is psychologically, as older bisexual people internalize these stereotypes. When bisexual people internalize biphobia, they are more likely to believe the stereotypes about bisexual people and to apply these stereotypes to themselves. The degree to which biphobic stereotypes are internalized is important, as it has consequences for health and mental health outcomes. Research indicates that bisexual individuals with higher degrees of internalized biphobia are more likely to demonstrate mental health challenges (Bostwick, 2012; Rothblum, Balsam, & Mickey, 2004). The internalization of biphobia may be one of the reasons that bisexual people experience the worst mental health outcomes (e.g., depression, anxiety, suicidality) when compared to heterosexual, lesbian, and gay individuals (Jorm et al., 2002).

Another challenge older bisexual people face is a sense of invisibility—a common experience for both older adults and bisexual people (Dworkin, 2006; Keppel & Firestein, 2007). The intersection of these identities may render bisexual older adults particularly invisible to helping professionals and other social contacts. For some bisexual people, this can emerge as people in their life make monosexist assumptions about their sexual orientation based on their gender identity and the gender identity of their partner (Scherrer, Kazyak, & Schmitz, 2015). For instance, a woman who is dating another woman is assumed to be lesbian or a man dating a woman is perceived to be heterosexual. Where for gay and lesbian people, one's relationship status often provides visibility for their identity in everyday life, bisexual people's relationship status may render their sexual orientation invisible. The issue of (in)visibility may be more complicated for older adults as their longer lives may have provided opportunities to introduce members of their social network to multiple significant others. For some older bisexual people, their longer lives may have afforded them additional opportunities for bisexual visibility.

Yet another complexity related to the invisibility of bisexuality for older adults emerges in an examination of cohort-related experiences in relationship to the concept of bisexuality (Rosenfield, 1999; Scherrer & Fedor, 2015). Although the concept of bisexuality has a long history in sexological scholarship, bisexuality did not garner public attention in the United States until the 1950s when Kinsey's research on the sexual practices of men and women conceptualized sexual orientation as existing on a continuum from exclusively heterosexual to exclusively homosexual (Rodriguez-Rust, 2002; Scherrer, 2013). The concept of bisexuality may have emerged from academic scholarship; however, it was activist movements of the 1960s and 70s that paved the way for bisexuality to demand inclusion alongside gay and lesbian sexual identities in social and political advocacy efforts. The 1980s ushered in a proliferation of books, magazines, conferences, and political groups pertaining to bisexuality (Rodriguez-Rust, 2002; Udis-Kessler, 1996) and brought a new level of visibility to this identity. In this way, the term bisexual has only recently become *culturally available* to adopt as an identity. Because of this history, older adults who grew up before the 1980s are likely to have spent more of their lives being unaware about bisexuality. Older adults with attraction to men and women may be reluctant to adopt a bisexual identity, based on its cultural availability during much of their life course, which may in turn make bisexual-identified older adults feel even more invisible. Thus, the intersection of sexual orientation and cohort membership influences older adults' comfort with and adoption of the identity label of bisexuality.

Recent scholarship on bisexuality in older adulthood indicates that some older adults are adopting a bisexual identity later in life. For example, when long-term relationships end, older adults may wish to explore same-sex desires they have kept quiet about earlier in life. Similarly, the more recent cultural availability of bisexual identities may make adopting a bisexual identity in later life more possible for older adults. Adopting a bisexual identity in later life can be a challenge as bisexual older adults may experience Dissonance of Stages of Development (DoSD) as their broader developmental activities are "out of line" with their sexual identity development, which more typically occurs in adolescence (Keppel & Firestein, 2007). Keppel and Firestein (2007) indicate that older adults, who are most likely engaged in the developmental task of generativity, or by giving back to the community and future generations, may experience dissonance in also undergoing a developmental task most frequently associated with younger adulthood (identity development). Keppel and Firestein (2007) posit that this developmental incongruence may produce challenges for older bisexual people, such as not having other peers to talk with about their sexual or relational interests and may further intensify feelings of invisibility and isolation.

Another way these stereotypes may present challenges is when bisexual older adults seek social support or community. For instance, like gay and lesbian people, bisexual people often experience homophobia (as well as biphobia) from heterosexual people in their social milieu. While gay and lesbian people often find safe havens from homophobia among other gay and lesbian people, this source of support and community is more fraught for bisexual people, as biphobic beliefs are widespread among gay and lesbian communities (McLean, 2008; Ochs, 1996). Indeed, bisexual people experience less social and familial support than their gay or lesbian counterparts (Jorm et al., 2002). These challenges play out not only with friends and other members of a bisexual person's social network, but they may also emerge in romantic relationships. Bisexual people may feel as though they cannot be their whole, authentic selves in friendships or romantic relationships with both heterosexual and/or lesbian/gay people. The lack of community and social support may be of particular import in working with bisexual *older adults* who are already vulnerable to issues of loneliness and isolation by virtue of their status as older adults (Keppel & Firestein, 2007).

Similar to their unique circumstances in finding community, bisexual people also experience unique challenges in their relationships with families

(McLean, 2007; Scherrer & Fedor, 2015; Scherrer, Kazyak, & Schmitz, 2015). Although little is known about bisexual people's experiences coming out to families of origin for any age group, nascent research on this topic indicates that stereotypes about bisexuality impact the strategies that bisexual people adopt when "coming out" to their family members (Scherrer, Kazyak, & Schmitz, 2015). Family members' responses to learning about a bisexual family members' sexual orientation are also shaped by stereotypes about bisexuality, for instance as family members may believe that bisexuality is a transitory identity on the way to a stable monosexual orientation (Scherrer, et al., 2015). In one salient example from a 55-year-old bisexual man who came out later in life, Scherrer et al. (2015) discuss how "Ralph's" faith community, who he described as his family, offered comfort to his wife after he came out because they assumed that "Ralph" would most likely be ending their relationship in favor of dating men. This example illustrates how biphobic stereotypes shape the ways that families and communities may interpret older adults' bisexuality, even in the context of a long-term marriage relationship.

Another challenge faced by bisexual older adults emerges in interactions with service providers. When discussing individual level interventions in this chapter, the words practitioner, service provider, and human service professional are used interchangeably to indicate a person working with a bisexual older adult client in a professional capacity (e.g., social worker, counselor, health provider, geriatric care manager). For bisexual people who are working with service providers, they may be challenged by practitioners' own problematic attitudes about bisexuality. For instance, practitioners' attitudes about bisexuality largely overlap with dominant cultural stereotypes about bisexuality (Eliason & Hughes, 2004; Mohr, Israel, & Sedlacek, 2001; Mohr et al., 2009; Page, 2007) and tend to be more negative toward bisexual people than to gay or lesbian clients (Eliason & Hughes, 2004). Furthermore, these attitudes shape interactions between bisexual clients and service providers. Research indicates that biphobic beliefs are correlated with more negative reactions to bisexual clients (Mohr, Israel, & Sedlacek, 2001), and practitioners imagine that stereotypes about bisexuality are relevant to client's problems (Mohr et al., 2009). Research also demonstrates that practitioners are more likely to negatively assess client functioning and the seriousness of the problem for bisexual clients, as well as practitioners' feelings about working with the client (Bowers & Bieschke, 2005; Mohr et al., 2009; Murphy, Rawlings, & Howe, 2002). Considering the vulnerability that both bisexual people and older adults contend with in contemporary society, it is critical that helping service professionals are well-trained to work in culturally competent capacities with bisexual older adults. The next section provides an overview of current research on best practices that pertain to bisexual older adults.

BEST PRACTICES FOR PRACTICE, PROGRAMS, AND POLICY

A small, but fruitful body of scholarship provides insight into how service providers may better support bisexual older adults in multiple levels of practice (Dworkin, 2006; Keppel, 2006; Keppel & Firestein, 2007; Rodriguez-Rust, 2012). The vast majority of previous scholarship on bisexual older adults has focused on how individual level interventions may be adapted to be more culturally competent in working with bisexual older adults, providing important insights into best practices for working with this community. One such practice strategy invites practitioners to seek out inclusive language when working with clients. Keppel (2006) suggests that inclusive language, such as when discussing the gender of current or previous partners or in privileging the client's own definition about who constitutes their family, may signify to a bisexual older adult client that a practitioner may be knowledgeable about monosexist assumptions. Similarly, using the word bisexual when asking about the client's sexual orientation may also help to signify a practitioner's cultural competence in working with bisexual clients (Keppel & Firestein, 2007).

Some bisexual older adults may seek support surrounding their sexual orientation, particularly those who have come to their identity later in life. Bisexual older adults who have come out later in life may benefit from awareness about bisexuality itself as well as about bisexual communities (Keppel & Firestein, 2007). Bisexual older adults may appreciate opportunities to strategize about how family and friends may respond to learning about their bisexuality, and it may be helpful to discuss how homophobia and biphobia may emerge in the reactions of friends and family. Although some bisexual older adults may seek out support around identity development, it is also important to note that for many, the presenting problems of bisexual older adults may have very little to do with their sexual orientation. Practitioners should be careful not to assume that the client's bisexuality is a problem in and of itself (Scherrer, 2013).

Practitioners must be aware of the history of bisexuality in contemporary society and demonstrate thoughtfulness about how the cultural availability of this identity label may have shaped an individual bisexual client's relationship to this identity. Being knowledgeable about social and historical context, vis-à-vis sexuality, will assist practitioners in recognizing cohort-related differences within populations of older adults. For instance, someone who came into adulthood during the 1930s and lived in a time period where it was common to use drastic measures to "treat" the "illness" of homosexuality may have been more likely to "pass" as heterosexual (Keppel & Firestein, 2007). In contrast, younger cohorts of older adults were more likely to have come to adulthood in a social context where Kinsey's research on human sexuality was well-publicized, where urban communities for individuals with same-sex desire were more established following the conclusion of World War II, and where there was a burgeoning effort of social and cultural activism for civil rights of marginalized communities (D'Emilio, 1983; Keppel & Firestein, 2007). For clients who come to their sexual identity later in life, they may be more likely to see bisexuality as a possible identity, based on bisexual activist communities during the 1980s and 90s. Being aware of how social and historical context may differentially shape older adults' views about sexual orientation, and bisexuality specifically, will assist practitioners in providing culturally competent services for bisexual older adults. Practitioners may wish to ask clients about how they were affected by these historical events and "what memories and fears they still carry with them" (Keppel & Firestein, 2007, p. 175).

It can be a challenge to find bisexual community at any age; however, this is likely to be especially challenging for bisexual older adults. As discussed previously, gay/lesbian older adult communities may not always be welcoming to bisexual older adults, and many bisexual communities, when they do exist, are often populated by younger bisexual people, which can be a challenge for bisexual older adults seeking social support based on sexual orientation (Dworkin, 2006). Trust will be a critical component for older bisexual adults' abilities to locate or create bi-affirming communities. Internet-based communities and online resources can be a potential resource for bisexual older adults in need of bisexual community and social support. However, practitioners must be thoughtful in making sure that their clients are comfortable using these resources (Keppel & Firestein, 2007). Clients may need encouragement and support in adopting new technologies to make use of these resources.

Practitioners should also seek out continuing education and support about working with bisexual older adult clients, potentially by creating such opportunities in their communities. As previously discussed, there is a lack of adequate training on issues related to bisexuality, even among those with knowledge about lesbian and gay populations (Mohr, Israel, & Sedlacek, 2001; Murphy, Rawlings, & Howe, 2002). Furthermore, there is a lack of training in working with bisexual people more generally (Mohr, Israel, & Sedlacek, 2001; Murphy, Rawlings, & Howe, 2002; Scherrer, 2013). In light of this research, practitioners should seek out additional opportunities to assess their own unconscious biases about bisexuality (Scherrer, 2013). In further consideration of the unique challenges that bisexual older adults face, trainings about bisexuality should seek to incorporate an intersectional lens in examining how identities such as race, gender, class, and most critically to this analysis, *age* and *cohort*, shape practitioners' work with bisexual clients.

On a programmatic level, service providers should strive to ensure that intake forms, assessment tools, descriptions of services on pamphlets and websites, and other organizational materials are inclusive of, and welcoming to, bisexual individuals. For example, forms should include bisexuality as an option in demographic forms that ask about clients' sexual orientation. Practitioners or organizations may display the bisexual flag or other images that promote visibility for bisexual people in their organizational space. Social service programs can also work to promote visibility of bisexuality within programs that work with the GLBT community as a means of supporting bisexual older adults (Keppel, 2006). For example, organizations can host events that focus specifically on issues relevant to bisexual older adults (e.g., visibility, community building, coming out to partners, family, friends) instead of simply including bisexuality as part of a discussion on lesbian and gay identities. As myriad scholars point out, bisexual people are often grouped together with lesbian and gay identities without any substantive analysis about potential within group differences, leaving attendees inadequately prepared to address the unique challenges of this population.

Social service interventions and programs that serve bisexual older adults (which arguably are all programs that serve older adults or GLBT populations) should capitalize on the resilience that bisexual people have often been required to cultivate, for instance as they navigate biphobia from heterosexual as well as gay/lesbian communities. Practitioners should seek out opportunities to affirm this strength and resilience with individual clients and develop programs that capitalize on these internal resources. Social service programs should develop a list of resources for bisexual older adults, which could include materials such as print or online educational content, contact information for relevant community groups, and media such as books, films or magazines.

CONCLUSION AND FUTURE DIRECTIONS

The lack of empirical research focusing on the experiences of bisexual older adults makes it almost trite to say that further research is needed on this population. There are a number of practical reasons for this paucity of research. First, small sample sizes limit bisexual-specific analyses of quantitative data that incorporate older GLBT individuals. Second, it may be that there are relatively few older adults who self-identify as bisexual, although demographic research on GLB identities would challenge this notion (Egan, Edelman, & Sherrill, 2007;

Hebenick et al., 2010; Mosher, Chandra, & Jones, 2005). While these challenges are considerable, the following are possible strategies to consider in moving forward empirical research on bisexual older adults. First, publishers, editors, and researchers should consider relaxing sample-size expectations for this hidden population and seek descriptive and demographic data about bisexual older adults. Second, researchers should seek to supplement sampling strategies to purposively include older bisexual participants, for instance by targeting bisexual communities when recruiting for research on GLBT populations. Third, much can be learned from qualitative research with small samples of older bisexual individuals. Researchers may wish to pursue qualitative data collection from this community as a means of building empirical and theoretical knowledge about this identity group.

Theoretical and practice-based scholarship has been more fruitful in extending knowledge about bisexual older adults (Dworkin, 2006; Keppel, 2006; Keppel & Firestein, 2007; Rodriguez-Rust, 2012). As discussed in this review, bisexual older adults experience unique challenges in social life, often related to biphobic attitudes. Although research often includes bisexual identities alongside lesbian and gay identities, bisexual people experience unique challenges. Thus, future research on sexual minority older adults should treat these identity categories as distinct and focus on differences that exist between gay, lesbian, and bisexual older adults. Furthermore, future research should also seek to examine diversity within populations of bisexual adults, as race, gender, age, and cohort have all been identified as characteristics that intersectionally shape bisexual people's lives.

In consideration of the challenges bisexual older adults face in light of stereotypes about older adults and bisexual people, further research should examine how these dissonant stereotypes play out in the lives of bisexual older adults. Future research may also fruitfully examine how biphobic stereotypes are internalized by bisexual older adults, particularly in relationships to their coming out process (e.g., coming out as bisexual earlier in life or later in life). It may be that timing of coming to a bisexual identity provides additional (or fewer) opportunities to challenge harmful stereotypes and develop resilience. Related to this, future research may also seek to examine how age and cohort shape bisexual people's mental health statuses. While literature has examined bisexual people's decision-making process around adopting a bisexual identity, less is known about how these identity adoption processes may be similar or different for older bisexual people—an issue that may be shaped by the cultural availability of sexual identity categories.

Scholarship indicates that invisibility is an issue for bisexual people of many age groups, yet little is known about what types of visibility bisexual older adults specifically may prefer. Related to issues of invisibility are the challenges that bisexual older adults face in regard to social and familial support. Little is known about older bisexual people's coming out experiences in families of origin, experiences in forming intimate relationships or constructing chosen families. Similarly, little is known about the unique strengths or challenges bisexual older adults demonstrate in their family lives. Finding social support and community may be a particular need of, and challenge for, bisexual older adults, and future research could fruitfully examine the types of communities or support services older bisexual adults would prefer. Another domain for possible future research is in developing trainings for geriatric service providers as well as for organizations that work with GLBT populations, to provide education about bisexual older adults (and bisexuality more generally).

If bisexuality is a very invisible identity in contemporary U.S. society, then older bisexual people are practically invisible. Moving forward there is great opportunity, and great need, to capitalize on rapidly increasing populations of older adults to better understand the diverse experiences of older adults. Employing an intersectional approach to understand the needs of bisexual older adults, GLBT people, and older adults more generally, provides much promise to understand the rich diversity and complexities of these communities. Gerontologists, sexuality scholars, practitioners, policy makers, researchers, and other professionals should all be invested in extending our knowledge about bisexual older adults so that we can better serve this marginalized and often invisible population.

REFERENCES

Barker, M., Bowes-Catton, H., Iantaffi, A., Cassidy, A., & Brewer, L. (2008). British bisexuality: A snapshot of bisexual identities in the United Kingdom. *Journal of Bisexuality*, *8*(1–2), 141–162.

Bertsch, K. N. (2014). *The relationship among anti-bisexual discrimination experiences and coping on bisexual women and men's mental health* (Unpublished doctoral dissertation). Lehigh University, Bethlehem, PA.

Bostwick, W. (2012). Assessing bisexual stigma and mental health status: A brief report. *Journal of Bisexuality, 12*(2), 214–222.

Bowers, A. M., & Bieschke, K. J. (2005). Psychologists' clinical evaluations and attitudes: An examination of the influence of gender and sexual orientation. *Professional Psychology: Research and Practice, 36*, 97–103.

Bowleg, L. (2012). The problem with the phrase women and minorities: Intersectionality-an important theoretical framework for public health. *American Journal of Public Health*, *102*(7), 1267–1273.

Bradford, M. (2004). The bisexual experience: Living in a dichotomous culture. *Journal of Bisexuality*, 4(1–2), 7–23.

Cohler, B. J. (2005). Life course social science perspectives on the GLBT family. *Journal of GLBT Family Studies, 1*(1), 69–95.

Collins, P. H. (2000). *Black feminist thought: Knowledge, consciousness and the politics of empowerment*. New York, NY: Routledge, Chapman and Hall.

D'Emilio, J. (1983). Capitalism and gay identity. In A. Snitow, C. Stansell, & S. Thompson (Eds.), *Powers of desire: The politics of sexuality* (pp. 100–113). New York, NY: Monthly Review Press.

Dodge, B., & Sandfort, T. (2007). A review of mental health research on bisexual individuals when compared to homosexual and heterosexual individuals. In B. Firestein (Ed.), *Becoming visible: Counseling bisexuals across the lifespan* (pp. 28–51). New York, NY: Columbia University Press.

Dworkin, S. (2006). The aging bisexual: The invisible of the invisible minority. In D. Kimmel, T. Rose, & S. David (Eds.), *Lesbian, gay, bisexual and transgender aging: Research and clinical perspectives* (pp. 36–52). New York, NY: Columbia University Press.

Egan, P. J., Edelman, M. S., & Sherrill, K. (2007). *Findings from the Hunter College Poll of Lesbians, Gays, and Bisexuals: New discoveries about identity, political attitudes, and civic engagement*. Hunter College, CUNY. Retrieved from http://as.nyu.edu/docs/IO/4819/hunter_college_poll.pdf

Eliason, M. (2001). Bi-negativity: The stigma facing bisexual men. *Journal of Bisexuality, 19*(2–3), 137–154.

Eliason, M. J., & Hughes, T. (2004). Treatment counselor's attitudes about lesbian, gay, bisexual, and transgendered clients: Urban vs. rural settings. *Substance use and Misuse, 39*, 625–644.

Esterberg, K. (2006). The bisexual menace revisited; or shaking up social categories is hard to do. In S. Seidman, N. Fisher, & C. Meeks (Eds.), *Handbook of the new sexuality studies: Original essays and interviews* (pp. 169–176). New York, NY: Routledge Press.

Goetstouwers, L. (2006). Affirmative psychotherapy with bisexual men. *Journal of Bisexuality*, 6(1–2), 27–49.

Hebenick, D., Reece, M., Schick, V., Sanders, S. A., Dodge, B., & Fortenberry, J. D. (2010). Sexual behavior in the United States: Results from a national probability sample of men and women aged 14–94. *Journal of Sexual Medicine*, 7, 255–265.

Henderson, L. (2009). Between the two: Bisexual identity among African Americans. *Journal of African American Studies, 13*, 263–282.

Herek, G. M. (2002). Heterosexuals' attitudes toward bisexual men and women in the United States. *Journal of Sex Research, 39*, 264–274.

Hodson, D., & Skeen, P. (1994). Sexuality and aging: The hammerlock of myths. *Journal of Applied Gerontology, 13*, 219–235.

Horowitz, J. L., & Newcomb, M. D. (1999). Bisexuality, not homosexuality: Counseling issues and treatment approaches. *Journal of College Counseling*, 2, 148–163.

Israel, T., & Mohr, J. J. (2004). Attitudes toward bisexual women and men: Current research, future direction. *Journal of Bisexuality, 4*(1–2), 117–134.

Jorm, A. F., Korten, A. E., Rodgers, B., Jacomb, P. A., & Christensen, H. (2002). Sexual orientation and mental health: Results from a community survey of young and middle-aged adults. *British Journal of Psychiatry, 180*, 423–427.

Keppel, B. (2006). Affirmative psychotherapy with older bisexual women and men. *Journal of Bisexuality*, 6(1–2), 85–104.

Keppel, B., & Firestein, B. (2007). Bisexual inclusion in addressing GLBT aging. In B. Firestein (Ed.), *Becoming visible: Counseling bisexuals across the lifespan* (pp. 164–185). New York, NY: Columbia University Press.

Kertzner, R., Meyer, I. H., Frost, D. M., & Stirratt, M. J. (2009). Social and psychological well-being in lesbians, gay men, and bisexuals: The effects of race, gender, age and sexual identity. *American Journal of Orthopsychiatry*, *79*, 500–510.

Kimmel, D., Rose, T., & David, S. (2006). *Lesbian, gay, bisexual and transgender aging: Research and clinical perspectives.* New York, NY: Columbia University Press.

Malebranche, D. J., Arriola, K., Jenkins, T. R., Dauria, E., & Patel, S. (2010). Exploring the "bisexual bridge": A qualitative study of risk behavior and disclosure of same-sex behavior among black bisexual men. *American Journal of Public Health, 100*, 159–164.

McLean, K. (2007). Hiding in the closet? Bisexual, coming out and the disclosure imperative. *Journal of Sociology, 43*, 151–166.

McLean, K. (2008). Inside, outside, nowhere: Bisexual men and women in the gay and lesbian community. *Journal of Bisexuality, 8*(1–2), 63–80.

Mohr, J., Israel, T., & Sedlacek, W. E. (2001). Counselors' attitudes regarding bisexuality as predictors of counselors' clinical responses: An analogue study of a female bisexual client. *Journal of Counseling Psychology*, *48*, 212–222.

Mohr, J., Weiner, J. L., Chopp, R. M., & Wong, S. J. (2009). Effects of client bisexuality on clinical judgment: When is bias most likely to occur? *Journal of Counseling Psychology*, *56*, 164–175.

Mosher, W. D., Chandra, A., & Jones, J. (2005). *Sexual behavior and selected health measures: Men and women 15–44 years of age, United States, 2002*. Atlanta, GA: US Department of Health and Human Services, Centers for Disease Control and Prevention, National Center for Health Statistics.

Murphy, J. A., Rawlings, E. I., & Howe, S. R. (2002). A survey of clinical psychologists on treating lesbian, gay, and bisexual clients. *Professional Psychology: Research and Practice, 33*, 183–189.

Ochs, R. (1996). Biphobia: It goes more than two ways. In B. A. Firestein (Ed.), *Bisexuality: The psychology and politics of an invisible minority* (pp. 217–239). Thousand Oaks, CA: Sage Publications.

Orel, N. A., & Fruhauf, C. A. (2014). *The lives of lesbian, gay, bisexual, and transgender (LGBT) older adults: Understanding challenges and resilience*. Washington, DC: American Psychological Association.

Page, E. (2007). Bisexual women's and men's experiences of psychotherapy. In B. Firestein (Ed.), *Becoming visible: Counseling bisexuals across the lifespan* (pp. 52–71). New York, NY: Columbia University Press.

Rodriguez-Rust, P. (2002). Bisexuality: The state of the union. *Annual Review of Sex Research, 13,* 180–240.

Rodriguez-Rust, P. (2012). Aging in the bisexual community. In T. Witten & A. E. Eyler (Eds.), *Gay, lesbian, bisexual and transgender aging: Challenges in research, practice and policy* (pp. 162–186). Baltimore, MD: Johns Hopkins University Press.

Rosenfield, D. (1999). Identity work among lesbian and gay elderly. *Journal of Aging Studies, 13*(2), 121–144.

Rothblum, E. D., Balsam, K. F., & Mickey, R. M. (2004). Brothers and sisters of lesbians, gay men, and bisexuals as a demographic comparison group: An innovative research methodology to examine social change. *Journal of Applied Behavioral Science, 40*, 283–301.

Scherrer, K. S. (2009). Images of sexuality and aging. *Sexuality Research and Social Policy, 6*(4), 5–12.

Scherrer, K. S. (2013). Clinical practice with bisexual identified individuals. *Clinical Social Work Journal, 41*(3), 238–248.

Scherrer, K. S., & Fedor, J. (2015). Family issues for LGBT older adults. In N. A. Orel & C. A. Fruhauf (Eds.), *The lives of lesbian, gay, bisexual, and transgender (LGBT) older adults: Understanding challenges and resilience* (pp. 171–192). Washington, DC: American Psychological Association.

Scherrer, K. S., Kazyak, E. A., & Schmitz, R. (2015). Getting 'bi' in the family: Bisexual people's disclosure strategies within the family. *Journal of Marriage and Family, 77*(3), 680–696.

Spalding, L. R., & Peplau, L. (1997). The unfaithful lover: Heterosexuals' stereotypes of bisexuals and their relationships. *Psychology of Women Quarterly, 21*, 611–625.

Udis-Kessler, A. (1996). Identity/Politics: Historical sources of the bisexual movement. In B. Beemyn & M. Eliason (Eds.), *Queer studies: A lesbian, gay, bisexual and transgender anthology* (pp. 52–63). New York, NY: University Press.

Witten, T., & Eyler, A. (2012). *Gay, lesbian, bisexual and transgender aging: Challenges in research, practice and policy*. Baltimore, MD: Johns Hopkins University Press.

Worth, H. (2003). The myth of the bisexual infector? *Journal of Bisexuality, 3*(2), 69–88.

CHAPTER 5

Mental Health for Older LGBT Adults

Shawn D. King and Virginia E. Richardson

ABSTRACT

This chapter examines the mental health of older lesbian, gay, bisexual, and transgender (LGBT) adults. Studies indicate higher levels of depression, suicide, and substance abuse among older LGBT adults compared to older heterosexual adults. Historical influences including outdated views of homosexuality as a mental illness especially affected the current cohort of older LGBT persons who also have been less likely to disclose their sexual identities. These issues as well as best practices, specifically Gay Affirmative Therapy, and core competencies needed when working with older LGBT adults are discussed in this chapter.

INTRODUCTION

Mental health is a part of one's overall health and quality of life influenced by and relating and interacting with physical health (World Health Organization, 2014). Although older LGBT people make up a substantial number of the estimated LGBT population overall, experts know little about older LGBT persons' mental health. Many issues make the study of mental health among older LGBT persons unique, including: (a) ageism and discrimination based on gender identity; (b) harassment and violence; and (c) unfriendly policies and services (Hash & Rogers, 2013). Hash and Rogers (2013) outline the consequences of

http://dx.doi.org/10.1891/0198-8794.37.59

lifelong discrimination especially in health care, caregiving, retirement policies, and end-of-life decisions, which have inevitably resulted in increased stress, more avoidance of preventative health care, and decreased access to health and mental health care for these older adults. Not surprisingly, many older LGBT feel "twice hidden" (Hash & Rogers, 2013). Blando (2001) and Schope (2005) have argued that ageism combined with discrimination about sexual orientation has marginalized many older LGBT persons and adversely influenced their well-being. These factors have also contributed to obfuscation in the research on older LGBT persons' mental health, especially when investigators fail to consider cohort and historical influences (Grendron, Pendleton, & White, 2016; Hash & Rogers, 2013).

Older LGBT individuals are a diverse group. They vary depending on the age cohort to which they belong and with respect to their race and ethnicity, gender, socioeconomic status, and geographic residence. For these reasons, this chapter is organized into two parts. In the first part, the mental health of older LGBT adults in general along with important influences on mental health, specifically, age cohort, income, social supports, and race and ethnicity is discussed. Within group variability is addressed in the second part by focusing on four subgroups: older gay men, older lesbians, older bisexual adults, and older transgender persons.

MENTAL HEALTH OF OLDER LGBTS

Despite some inconsistent results, most scholars have found higher levels of mental distress, including substance abuse, depression, loneliness, and suicide, among older LGBT adults compared to their same age peers who identify as heterosexual (Cochran & Mays, 2000; de Vries, 2014; Fredriksen-Goldsen, Kim, Barkan, Muraco, & Hoy-Ellis, 2013; Hash & Rogers, 2013; King et al., 2007; Wallace et al., 2011). Gendron and colleagues (2016) argue that older LGBT persons are especially at risk for depression because of their lifelong exposure to stigma, discrimination, and victimization resulting from their sexual orientation and/or gender identity. In addition, older LGBT adults are more likely to live alone and have no children (de Vries, 2014). Although results consistently show more mental distress among older LGBT adults than among older non-LGBT elderly persons, when confounding influences such as age, cohort, income, social supports, culture, minority stress, and coping styles are taken into account the results are more complex.

COHORT EFFECTS

Age cohort is perhaps the most important variable that is confounded with mental distress among this population. For example, in a cross-sectional survey of older LGBT adults, Fredriksen-Goldsen, Kim, Shiu, Goldsen, and Emlet (2015) found that mental health quality of life was highest for the middle-old cohort (between the ages of 65 and 79) and similar between the young-old (between 50 and 64) and the old-old (80 and older) age groups. They also found that victimization and discrimination were higher for the young-old and old-old age groups than for the middle-aged group. Perhaps the most important issue is that because scholars report that older LGBT persons are substantially less likely to disclose their sexual identities it becomes almost impossible for researchers to study and for practitioners to support these older adults. Longitudinal studies that control for age cohort differences among older LGBT adults are especially needed.

These cohort differences are due to many factors, but most likely are due to historical changes related to the discrimination of LGBT individuals. For example, the current cohort of LGBT persons over the age of 65 has aged in a society that has viewed them as mentally ill with a "sociopathic personality disorder" that needed treatment. This view dominated the ideology about homosexuality within society, including the medical world, until it was removed from the *Diagnostic and Statistical Manual of Mental Disorders* in 1973. Older LGBT persons often were subjected to cruel treatment including castration, lobotomies, reparative therapy treatments, being involuntary institutionalized, and other brutalities (Fredriksen-Goldsen, Cook-Daniels, et al., 2014; Silverstein, 2009).

MINORITY STRESS

Exposure to minority stressors, such as victimization and discrimination, also has influenced mental health among older LGBT adults. Several researchers (e.g., Cochran, Sullivan, & Mays, 2003; Wright, Owen, & Catalan, 2012; King & Richardson, in press), have shown that when a person who has a minority sexual identity is subjected to multiple minority stress factors, such as stigma, anticipation of stigma, and discrimination, they often experience more mental health distress. Gendron et al. (2016) and Fredriksen-Goldsen et al. (2013) also have found worse mental health outcomes among those who reported more victimization earlier in life. D'Augelli, Grossman, Hershberger, and O'Connell (2001) reported that about 75% of their sample of older LGBT adults reported some form of victimization. When LGBT persons are forced to conceal their sexual orientation to avoid discrimination and the stigma associated with being gay, which was more common among the older cohort, they can experience internalized homonegativity, which inevitably exacerbates mental distress. Such trauma often persists, remaining intractable to societal changes in legislation or in attitudes about homosexuality.

INCOME AND OTHER PROTECTIVE FACTORS

While some influences, such as minority stress, heighten mental distress, others buffer adversity. For example, several researchers, such as D'Augelli et al. (2001) and Fredriksen-Goldsen et al. (2015), have found that high income has a favorable impact on older LGBT adults' mental health. Older LGBT persons who have more social resources, including broad social networks and "families of choice," are also less likely to be depressed than those who remain socially isolated (Fredriksen-Goldsen et al., 2015).

Other protective factors that researchers have identified include high self-esteem and self-efficacy, a strong sense of agency, and emotional control (Gralinski-Bakker, Hauser, Stott, Billings, & Allen, 2004; Luthar, Chicchetti, & Becker, 2000). These protective factors underlie resilient aging, which has become increasingly emphasized in the gerontology literature and linked to positive well-being, strong mental health, and competent functioning in work and interpersonal relationships (Gralinski-Bakker et al., 2004). More recently, it has been used as a model for understanding older LGBT persons' mental health (Fredriksen-Goldsen et al., 2015; King & Orel, 2012). Dentato and colleagues (2014) found that older LGBT adults who had access to these protective factors resembled what Fry and Keyes (2010, p. 3) have defined as resilient aging, which is:

> The need for individuals to strike a healthy balance between accumulating and preserving valued sources of life-strengths and related psychosocial resources for the future, and using valuable resources to deal with important needs in the present.

INTERSECTIONALITY: INTRACATEGORICAL INVESTIGATIONS

Until recently, most researchers have compared older LGBT adults' mental health to their heterosexual counterparts. While similarities as well as differences have been observed between these populations, gerontologists now recognize the diversity within the older LGBT population. According to Fish (2008, paragraph 2.3),

> Although there has been some success in identifying LGBT as a social category, the focus on inter-group differences (that is between LGBT people and their heterosexual counterparts) has occluded intra-group differences (that is differences within LGBT as an inequality category, for example in terms of race, disability and age).

Intersectionality scholars, for example, Murphy, Hunt, Zajicek, Norris, and Hamilton (2009), typically eschew a homogenized understanding of older LGBT individuals and instead value the diversity, nuances, and complexities within subgroups. For example, Fish (2008) applied an intersectionality framework to examine how class and gender influenced lesbians' experiences and how racism and heterosexism intersected in the lives of gay men. Findings from studies that have examined within group differences have mostly focused on: older gay men, older lesbians, older bisexual adults, and older transgender persons.

GAY MEN AND MENTAL HEALTH

Depression among older gay men is twice as common as it is among older heterosexual men (de Vries, 2014). Several scholars (e.g., Cahill & Valadez, 2013; de Vries, 2014; King & Orel, 2012; Wight, LeBlanc, deVries, & Detels, 2012) attribute the higher incidence of depression among gay men to their experiences with HIV/AIDS infection and the loss of many friends to this disease, referred to as HIV bereavement. HIV bereavement is unique given the untimeliness of deaths, nontraditional relationships, social isolation, uniqueness, the stigma associated with the disease, and disenfranchised grief (Jenkins, Edmundson, Avertt, & Yoon, 2014). According to Doka (1989), disenfranchised grief is associated with losses, such as miscarriages, abortions, suicides, divorces, that people experience that typically remain hidden from society and unacknowledged. Complicated grief reactions are more likely to occur under these circumstances especially when they preclude the social support more often following traditional bereavement events that are publicly noticed and mourned.

People with HIV/AIDS are living longer due to advancements in antiretroviral drugs than in the past. It is estimated that within 2 years, half of the 1.2 million Americans living with HIV will be 50 years old or older (King & Orel, 2012; High, Brennan-Ing, Clifford, Cohen, & Deeks, 2012). However, complications related to growing older with this disease have exacerbated mental distress among older gay men (Cahill & Valadez, 2013). For example, in a cross-sectional study of 316 midlife and older gay men, King and Orel (2012) found that midlife and older gay men living with HIV/AIDS more often reported suicidal thoughts, a diagnosis of substance dependency, and/or clinical depression compared to older gay men who were not living with HIV/AIDS. Wight and colleagues (2012) also examined the association between stress and mental health among 202 midlife and older gay men using data from the University of California, Los Angeles component of the Multicenter AIDS cohort study. They found several stressors, including sexual minority stress, stress associated with growing older, and loss associated with HIV bereavement have resulted in poor mental health among these men. The stigma related to HIV has also been linked to high mental distress and hesitation to seek help (Cahill & Valadez, 2013). Similarly, King and Richardson (in press) observed an association between discrimination due to sexual orientation and mental distress. They also found cohort effects. The younger midlife age cohort of gay men (those between the ages of 45 and 64) had higher levels of mental health distress than the older cohort of men (those 65 years old and older). Although older gay men have had to cope with lifelong struggles associated with minority stress, such as stigma, discrimination, and internalized homophobia, some experts, (e.g., David & Knight, 2008), argue that older gay men were forced to cope differently from younger gay men with these stressors. Kimmel (1978) calls these "crisis competency" skills.

Mental distress, including suicide ideation, also is higher among socially isolated gays than their more engaged peers. Those who have remained "in the closet" and still struggle with "coming out" are especially vulnerable (Cahill & Valadez, 2013; Cochran, Mays, Alegria, Ortega, & Takeuchi, 2007; Substance Abuse and Mental Health Services Administration, 2012; Wight et al., 2012). Older gay men who are partnered or legally married evidence better mental health outcomes than their unpartnered counterparts (Wright et al., 2012; King & Richardson, in press).

The few scholars who have examined the intersection between race and sexual identity underscore the unique challenges that Black gay and Black bisexual men have had to confront (Crawford, Allison, Zamboni, & Soto, 2002; Wilson, 2008; Wilson & Miller, 2002; Wilson et al., 2009). These include negative stereotypes about Black men and bisexual men; heterosexism within Black communities; and difficulties juggling multiple social identities. Bowleg (2013) interviewed 12 Black self-identified gay and bisexual men to examine the intersections of race and sexual identity, although the sample comprised men ranging in age from 21 to 44. Despite the lack of emphasis on older Black men, Bowleg's results are relevant. For example, she found that all but one of the 12 participants felt it was difficult to be Black men in general, and Black gay or bisexual men in particular. Their narratives revolved around four themes: (a) negative stereotypes about Black men or Black gay men; (b) racial microaggressions (i.e., subtle forms of racism) in mainstream and White LGB communities; (c) heterosexism in Black communities; and (d) the perceived pressure to act masculine to avoid suspicions of being gay or bisexual. Almost all mentioned their experiences of racism with White LGB communities. They felt that many White LGBs were uncomfortable with Black LGBs and expected them to assimilate and act like them. They often concealed their sexual identities, especially within the Black community. At the same time, several men reported benefits to being Black, gay, or bisexual men suggesting that their struggles promoted introspection, psychological growth, and freedom from social conventions. Bowleg (2013) challenged previous assumptions that multiple identities are simply additive rather than "mutually constituted." These participants felt they were unable to separate out one identity from another, although most felt that they were "Black first," suggesting some ranking of identities among these men. Bowleg (2013) also concluded that compared to traditional men these older men demonstrated greater resilience given the challenges they have had to confront throughout their lives. Her conclusions are consistent with those of Meyer, Dietrich, and Schwartz (2008) who found that Black LGBs had the lowest prevalence of lifetime mental disorders compared with White and Latino LGBs. Although the small sample size precludes us from generalizing from this research, these findings underscore the need for more research on these older men and the importance of recognizing the diversity within the subpopulation of older gay men and within the LGBT population in general.

LESBIAN MENTAL HEALTH

Older lesbians more often report depression than older heterosexual women (de Vries, 2014). However, when lesbians and bisexual women are compared, bisexual women evidence more mental distress, especially during midlife (Fredriksen-Goldsen, Kim, Barkan, Balsam, & Mincer, 2010). In general, Koh and Roh (2006) observed that the older lesbians who were at greatest risk for suicide and other mental health problems were not "out" and experienced a lot of emotional distress as teenagers. This finding is especially of concern given the research that has shown that many lesbians prefer to conceal their sexual identities (Substance Abuse and Mental Health Services Administration, 2012). With respect to substance abuse, older lesbians report more excessive drinking than older bisexual women (Fredriksen Goldsen et al., 2013).

Minority stress factors, specifically internalized homophobia, discrimination events, and the emotional distress some women associate with expressing masculine traits have been found to exacerbate mental health distress among lesbians (Nyitray, Corran, Altman, Chikani, & Negron, 2006). Social class differences have also been reported. Those with more socioeconomic resources, including education and income, have more options especially in their later years (Fish, 2008; McDermott, 2006). Experts however, have found that older lesbian women are more protected from ageism within their communities because they tend to have more social networks comprising lesbians from different age groups compared to their younger peers (Averett, Yoon, & Jenkins, 2011). They also tend to reject age-related and normative beauty standards and have generally benefited from the more positive views about aging that many in the feminist movement have supported. Younger lesbians often revere older lesbians for their wisdom and perceived political power (Schope, 2005).

In contrast to the research on older gay men, few studies have examined within group variability among older lesbian women. Future investigations need to examine potential buffers to mental health distress, such as being partnered, resilience, and social supports among older lesbian women given that these factors have been found to successfully mitigate the adverse impact of many minority stressors for older gay men.

BISEXUAL MENTAL HEALTH

Several investigators have found that when compared to older gays and lesbians, older bisexual adults evidence poorer mental health, and specifically more depression and anxiety (Dobinson, 2007; Fredriksen-Goldsen et al., 2011). Furthermore, Dobinson (2007) has reported that compared to heterosexuals, lesbians, and gay men, bisexuals are at greater risk for self-harm, and thoughts as well as attempts of suicide. Older bisexual individuals face many unique challenges that very likely contribute to their greater distress, although we need more studies on these older persons to better understand these issues.

Many bisexual persons feel they have been spurned by the gay and lesbian community for their more equivocal sexual identities (Hash & Rogers, 2013; Keppel, 2006). Based on results from Bowleg's (2013) research, these feelings might be especially common among Black and other ethnic minority LGBT older persons. Although bisexual persons are more likely to have been legally married, they still have sparser social networks compared to their gay or lesbian peers (Grossman, D'Augelli, & Herschberger, 2000). Fredriksen-Goldsen et al. (2011), found that compared to older lesbians, older bisexual women less often had a primary health care provider and more often feared seeking health care within the LGBT community at nearly three times the rate of older lesbian women. Older bisexual men also have unique issues. Although they are more likely to have children compared to their older gay peers, compared to heterosexual men, they are more likely to live alone (Fredriksen-Goldsen, 2011). Caregiving among bisexuals is also more often a combination of heterosexual and LGBT persons than it is among older lesbians or gay men (Travis & Kimmel, 2014).

In contrast to gay men and lesbians, bisexual adults are less likely to disclose their sexual minority identity to coworkers, neighbors, friends, and health care professionals, which is another factor that increases these older persons' social isolation, marginality, and mental distress (de Vries, 2014; Fredriksen-Goldsen et al., 2010; MetLife, 2010; Travis & Kimmel, 2014). Previous research has shown that concealment of one's sexual identity often causes more stress for bisexuals who must navigate multiple worlds in different contexts and at different times in their lives (Cant, 2005; Fish, 2008). According to Cass's (1979) model of identity formation, individuals who reveal and discuss their feelings about their sexual identities with those who accept them benefit in many ways compared to those who hide their identity. They benefit from opportunities to meet a partner; the provision of role models; and practice feeling more at ease with oneself as an LGBT person, which opens up potential to belong to a support group and achieve validation of the self as LGBT (Fish, 2008). At the same time, Fish (2008) argues that this characterization of "coming out" may be culturally and conceptually biased by relying on White, western constructs serving to pathologize the coming out experiences of Black and other ethnic minority LGBT persons. Fish purports that coming out as a lesbian or gay man might have serious negative consequences in some contexts. More research on bisexuals from diverse ethnic backgrounds is needed before conclusions about the benefits of "coming out" can be assumed for all subpopulations within the LGBT community.

TRANSGENDER MENTAL HEALTH

Mayer et al. (2008) define transgender as used exclusively to describe individuals who have "gender identities, expressions, or behaviors not traditionally associated with their birth sex" (p. 990). Only .3% to .5% of the population identify as transgender (Gates, 2011). Witten and Eyler (2012) believe the 65 and older transgender population to be approximately 700,000. Not surprisingly, they are the most underresearched group within the LGBT population, and most studies of the mental health of transgender persons have focused on younger cohorts (Institute of Medicine, 2011). In general, transgender persons have experienced the most abuse and been subjected to the most hate crimes of any LGBT subgroup (Grant et al., 2011; Witten & Eyler, 2012). Relative to the other subgroups, they have the poorest overall mental and physical health (Fredriksen-Goldsen, Cook-Daniels, et al., 2014). When Fredriksen-Goldsen et al. (2013) examined the types of discrimination and victimization transgender individuals experienced, they found that 76% reported verbal insults; 54% had been threatened with physical violence; 40% had been denied a job; 40% had inferior or were denied health care; 39% had not been promoted; and 37% had been treated inappropriately by police. These older persons also evidenced severe internalized stigma and more often concealed their gender identity compared to other LGB adults.

Transgender adults have the highest rates of depression of any LGBT subgroup (Clements-Nolle, Marx, Guzman, & Katz, 2001). Based on data from the Aging and Health Survey, Fredriksen-Goldsen et al. (2011) reported that 48% of older transgender adults compared to 31% of all LGBT individuals evidenced depression symptoms. Transgender individuals also have the highest rates of suicide ideation at 71% compared to 39% of all LGBT (Fredriksen-Goldsen et al., 2011). In addition, they also are high risks for suicide attempts

(Grant et al., 2011). Some studies have found that between 38% and 65% of these individuals have suicidal thoughts and between 16% and 32% have attempted suicide (Substance Abuse and Mental Health Services Administration, 2012). The few studies that have compared transgender men to transgender women have found that transgender women report more suicidal ideation, take more prescribed psychotropic medications, and experience more alcohol problems than transgender men. No differences have been found between lesbian and transgender women; however, transgender women evidence more depression and suicidal ideation than men who have sex with men and bisexual active women (Substance Abuse and Mental Health Services Administration, 2012). Transgender persons also have limited social supports, and they often feel rejected by the LGB community (Fredriksen-Goldsen et al., 2011; Grant et al., 2011). Fredriksen-Goldsen et al. (2013) found that compared to older gay men or older lesbians, transgender persons are more likely to have children and larger social networks but often find that their supports are inaccessible, which further exacerbates their mental health distress.

Despite the high need, older transgender adults are often denied services or face barriers to using services (Witten, 2014). These barriers include discrimination, lack of inclusion, strict gender guidelines in programs, and hostility and lack of empathy by health care providers (Substance Abuse and Mental Health Services Administration, 2012). Instead of getting help, older transgender adults more often feel harassed and victimized by their health care providers compared to other LGB adults (Grant et al., 2011). The lack of formal and informal support among transgender adults especially as they age is problematic given the high suicide rates, severe mental distress, and harassment these individuals experience over the life span. The inaccessibility of aging and end-of-life services to transgender old persons is evident in their reports of substantial fears about aging, death, and dying. Witten (2014) recently reported findings from a survey of 1,963 older persons that included the following identities: transsexual, transgender, intersex, disorders of sexual development, cross-gender, gender variant, gender-queer-identified, first nations, and non-Western gender identities. Among these transgender adults, 53% expressed concerns about how they would be cared for later in life, and few had made preparations for their retirement years. End-of-life discussions are difficult for anyone especially as they grow older, but transgender adults are especially vulnerable because their informal supports are more fragile and formal support systems remain inaccessible for many reasons, including lack of knowledge about older transgender persons and hesitations among these older adults to seek help from traditional service providers.

FUTURE DIRECTIONS AND BEST PRACTICES

In sum, older LGBT persons evidence more mental distress than their heterosexual peers while older bisexual and older transgender adults have more mental health problems than older gay men and lesbians. In addition, consistent with Meyer's minority stress theory, stigma, discrimination, and internalized homophobia each independently affect levels of psychological distress (Meyer, 1995; Meyer, 2003; Meyer, Dietrich, & Schwartz, 2008). When these stressors multiply and intersect, an older LGBT person's mental health inevitably worsens. More importantly, the unique issues characterizing subgroups of older LGBT individuals preclude us from generalizing about the overall older LGBT population especially when taking into account age cohort, minority stressors, and protective factors. Thus, a framework of intersectionality is preferred when researching these older adults and when providing them with services.

In addition to the need for more longitudinal and complex research designs that consider how multiple factors (e.g., age, cohort, gender, race and ethnicity, social class, geographic region) simultaneously influence people's lives over the life span, we also must follow best practices. For example, gay affirmative therapy (GAT), as articulated by Harrison (2000) and by Van Den Bergh and Crisp (2004), includes aspects of the person-in-environment and strengths-based perspective underlying cultural competency models (Crisp & McCave, 2007). In addition, GAT is based on intervention techniques that build self-esteem, view gay, lesbian, bisexual, and transgender individuals in a nonpathological manner, and center on increasing counselor understanding of those personal and professional barriers that would interfere with incorporating gay affirmative beliefs and attitudes into mental health therapeutic settings. Dillion and Worthington (2003) have identified crucial attitudes that mental health professionals, including psychologists, clinical social workers, and other counselors must adopt when implementing GAT. They include: focusing on the issues surrounding gay, lesbian, and bisexual individuals instead of viewing these issues from heterosexual norms that further marginalize this population; advocating the authenticity and integrity of lesbian, gay, and bisexual persons and their relationships; and understanding internalized homophobia and how other homophobic attitudes damage people's self-esteem.

GAT also is consistent with the core competencies that Fredriksen-Goldsen, Hoy-Ellis, et al. (2014) have identified that practitioners need to address when working with this population. These competencies include:

- Challenging heterosexism as the dominant culture's attitude as what is considered most natural and normal in human sexuality

- Knowing about the historical, social, and cultural forces that have marginalized and oppressed many LGBT persons and that have contributed to their mental distress
- Distinguishing similarities and differences within the subgroups of LGBT older adults; recognizing intersecting identities (such as age, gender, race, and health status)
- Understanding relevant conceptual perspectives, including the minority stress perspective, resilience, and intersectionality, that especially pertain to older LGBT adults
- Respecting the various structures of LGBT families as well as the importance of families of choice in providing instrumental, emotional, and social support
- Recognizing the ways that services can marginalize and discriminate against LGBT older persons
- Knowing ways to advocate for legislation on behalf of older LGBT adults at local, state, and federal levels
- Engaging in sensitive and appropriate outreach to LGBT older persons and their families

These competencies and best practices need to infiltrate not just our educational and social services infrastructures, but they also need to be acknowledged by various professionals in all settings if we expect to enhance mental health quality of life for all older persons regardless of their age, race, gender, or sexual identity.

REFERENCES

Averett, P., Yoon, I., & Jenkins, C. L. (2011). Older lesbians: Experiences of aging, discrimination and resilience. *Journal of Women and Aging, 23*, 216–232.

Blando, J. A. (2001). Twice hidden: Older gay and lesbian couples, friends, and intimacy. *Generations*, *25*(2), 87–89.

Bowleg, L. (2013). "Once you've blended the cake, you can't take the parts back to the main ingredients": Black gay and bisexual men's descriptions and experiences of intersectionality. *Sex Roles*, *68*(1/2), 754–767.

Cahill, S., & Valadez, R. (2013). Growing older with HIV/AIDS: New public health challenges. *American Journal of Public Health, 103*(3), E7–E15.

Cant, B. (2005). Exploring the implications for health professionals of men coming out as gay in healthcare settings. *Health and Social Care in the Community, 14*(1), 9–16.

Cass, V. C. (1979). Homosexual identity formation: A theoretical model. *Journal of Homosexuality*, *4*(3), 219–235.

Clements-Nolle, K., Marx, R., Guzman, R., & Katz, M. (2001). HIV prevalence, risk behaviors, health care use, and mental health status of transgender persons: Implications for public health intervention. *American Journal of Public Health, 91*(6), 915–921.

Cochran, S. D., & Mays, V. M. (2000). Lifetime prevalence of suicide symptoms and affective disorders among men reporting same-sex sexual partners: Results from NHANES III. *American Journal of Public Health*, *90*(4), 573–578.

Cochran, S. D., Mays, V. M., Alegria, M., Ortega, A. N., & Takeuchi, D. (2007). Mental health and substance abuse disorders among Latino and Asian American lesbian, gay, and bisexual adults. *Journal of Consulting and Clinical Psychology*, *75*(5), 785–794.

Cochran, S. D., Sullivan, J. G., & Mays, V. M. (2003). Prevalence of mental disorders, psychological distress, and mental health services use among lesbian, gay, bisexual adults in the United States. *Journal of Consulting and Clinical Psychology, 71*(1), 53–61.

Crawford, I., Allison, K. W., Zamboni, B. D., & Soto, T. (2002). The influence of dual-identity development on the psychosocial functioning of African-American gay and bisexual men. *Journal of Sex Research*, *39*, 179–189.

Crisp, C., & McCave, E. L. (2007). A model for social work practice with gay, lesbian, and bisexual youth. *Journal of Child Adolescent Social Work*, *24*, 403–421.

David, S., & Knight B. G. (2008). Stress and coping among gay men: and ethnic differences. *Psychology and Aging*, *23*, 62–69.

D'Augelli, A. R., Grossman, A. H., Hershberger, S. L., & O'Connell, T. S. (2001). Aspects of mental health among older lesbian, gay, and bisexual adults. *Aging and Mental Health*, *5*, 149–158.

Dentato, P., Orwat, J., Spira, M., & Walker, B. (2014). Examining cohort differences and resilience among the aging LGBT community: Implications for education and practice among an expansively diverse population. *Journal of Human Behavior in the Social Environment*, *24*, 316–328.

De Vries, B. (2014). LG (BT) persons in the second half of life: The intersectional influences of stigma and cohort. *LGBT Health*, *1*(1), 18–23.

Dillon, F. R., & Worthington, R. I. (2003). The lesbian, gay, and bisexual affirmative counseling self-efficacy inventory (LGB-CSI): Development, validation, and training implications. *Journal of Counseling Psychology, 50*(2), 235–251.

Dobinson, C. (2007). Top ten bisexual health issues. As cited in Miller, M., Andre, A., Ebin, J., & Bessonova, L. (2007). Bisexual health: An introduction and model practices for HIV/STI prevention programming. New York, NY: National Gay and Lesbian Task Force Policy Institute, The Fenway Institute at Fenway Community Health, and BiNet USA.

Doka, K. (1989). *Disenfranchised grief*. Lexington, MA: Lexington Books.

Fish, J. (2008). Navigating queer street: Researching the intersections of lesbian, gay, bisexual and Trans (LGBT) identities in health research. *Sociological Research Online*, *13*(1). Retrieved from http://www.socresonline.org.uk/13/1/12.html

Fredriksen-Goldsen, K. I., Cook-Daniels, L., Kim, H. J., Erosheva, E. A., Emlet, C. A., Hoy-Ellis, C. P., et al. (2014). Physical and mental health of transgender older adults: An at-risk and underserved population. *The Gerontologist, 54*, 488–500.

Fredriksen-Goldsen, K. I., Emlet, C. A., Kim, H. J., Muraco, A., Erosheva, E. A., Goldsen, J., & Hoy-Ellis, C. P. (2012). The physical and mental health of lesbian, gay male, and bisexual (LGB) older adults: The role of key health indicators and risk and protective factors. *The Gerontologist, 53*(4), 664–675.

Fredriksen-Goldsen, K. I., Hoy-Ellis, C. P., Goldsen, J., Emlet, C. A., & Hooyman N. R. (2014). Creating a vision for the future: Key competencies and strategies for culturally competent practice with lesbian, gay, bisexual, and transgender (LGBT) older adults in the health and human services. *Journal of Gerontological Social Work, 57*(2–4), 80–107.

Fredriksen-Goldsen, K. I., Kim, H. J., Barkan, S. E., Balsam, K. F., & Mincer, S. L. (2010). Disparities in health-related quality of life: A comparison of lesbians and bisexual women. *American Journal of Public Health, 100*(11), 2255–2261.

Fredriksen-Goldsen, K. I., Kim, H. J., Barkan, S. E., Muraco, A., & Hoy-Ellis, C. P. (2013). Health disparities among lesbian, gay male, and bisexual older adults: Results from a population-based study. *American Journal of Public Health, 103*, 1802–1809.

Fredriksen-Goldsen, K. I., Kim, H. J., Emlet, C. A., Muraco, A., Erosheva, E. A., Hoy-Ellis, C. P., et al. (2011). *The Aging and Health Report: Disparities and Resilience among Lesbian, Gay, Bisexual, and Transgender Older Adults.* Seattle, WA: Institute for Multigenerational Health. Retrieved from http://caringandaging.org

Fredriksen-Goldsen, K. I., Kim, H. J., Shiu, C., Goldsen, J., & Emlet, C. A. (2015). Successful aging among LGBT older adults: Physical and mental health-related quality of life by age group. *Gerontologist*, 55(1), 154–168.

Fry, P., & Keyes, C. L. M. (2010). Introduction. In Prem S. Fry & Corey L. M. Keyes (Eds.), *New frontiers in resilient aging: Life-strengths and well-being in late life* (pp. 1–14). Cambridge, UK: Cambridge University Press.

Gates, G. J. (2011). *How many people are lesbian, gay, bisexual, and transgender?* Los Angeles, CA: The Williams Institute.

Gralinski-Bakker, J. H., Hauser, S. T., Stott, C., Billings, R. L., & Allen, J. P. (2004). Markers of resilience and risk: Adult lives in a vulnerable population. *Research in Human Development, 1*(4), 291–326.

Grant, J. M., Mottet, L. A., Tanis, J., Harrison, J., Herman, J. L., & Keisling, M. (2011). *Injustice at every turn: A report of the national transgender discrimination survey.* Washington, DC: National Center for Transgender Equality and National Gay and Lesbian Task Force.

Gendron, T. L., Pendeton, T., & White, J. T. (2016). Mental health counseling of LGBT elders. In D. A. Harley & P. B. Teaster (Eds.), *Handbook of LGBT elders* (pp. 455–471). Switzerland: Springer Publishing.

Grossman, A. H., D'Augelli, A. R., & Hershberger, S. L. (2000). Social support networks of lesbian, gay, and bisexual adults 60 years of age and older. *Journal of Gerontology, Series B: Psychological Sciences, 55B*(3), P171–P179.

Harrison, N. (2000). Gay affirmative therapy: A critical analysis of the literature. *British Journal of Guidance and Counseling*, *28*(1), 37–53.

Hash, K M., & Rogers A. (2013). Clinical practice with older LGBT clients: Overcoming lifelong stigma through strength and resilience. *Clinical Social Work Journal*, *41*, 249–257.

High, K. P., Brennan-Ing, M., Clifford, D. B., Cohen, M. H., Currier, J., Deeks, S. G., & Volberding, P. (2012). HIV and aging: State of knowledge and areas of clinical need for research. A report to the NIH office of AIDS research by the HIV and aging working group. *Journal of Acquired Immune Deficiency Syndrome*, *60*, S1–S18.

Institute of Medicine. (2011). *The health of lesbian, gay, bisexual, and transgender people: Building a foundation for better understanding*. Washington, DC: The National Academies Press.

Jenkins, C. L., Edmundson, A., Averett, P., & Yoon, I. (2014). Older lesbians and bereavement: Experiencing the loss of a partner. *Journal of Gerontological Social Work*, *52*, 273–287.

Keppel, B. (2006). Affirmative psychotherapy with older bisexual women and men. *Journal of Bisexuality*, *6*(1/2), 85–104.

Kimmel, D. C. (1978). Adult development and aging: A gay perspective. *Journal of Social Issues*, *34*, 113–130.

King, S., & Orel, N. (2012). Midlife and older gay men living with HIV/AIDS: The influence of resiliency and psychosocial stress factors on health needs. *Journal of Gay and Lesbian Social Services*, *24*(4), 346–370.

King, S. D., & Richardson, V. E. (in press). Influence of income, being partnered/married, resiliency, and discrimination on mental health distress for midlife and older gay men. *Journal of Gay and Lesbian Mental Health*.

King, M., Semlyen, J., Tai, S. S., Killaspy, H., Osborn, D., Popelyuk, D., et al. (2007). A systematic review of mental disorder, suicide, and deliberate self harm in lesbian, gay and bisexual people. *BMC Psychiatry*, *8*(1), 70.

Koh, A. S., & Ross, L. K. (2006). Mental health issues: A comparison of lesbian, bisexual and heterosexual women. *Journal of Homosexuality*, *51*(1), 33–57.

Luthar, S. S., Chicchetti, D., & Becker, B. (2000). The construct of resilience. A critical evaluation and guidelines for future work. *Child Development*, *71*(3), 543–562.

Mayer, K. H., Bradford, J. B., Makadon, H. J., Stall, R., Goldhammer, H., & Landers, S. (2008). Sexual and gender minority health: What we know and what needs to be done. *American Journal of Public Health*, *98*(6), 989–995.

McDermott, E. (2006). Surviving in dangerous places: Lesbian identity performances in the workplace, social class, and psychological health. *Feminism and Psychology*, *16*(2), 193–211.

MetLife. (2010). *Still Out, Still Aging: The Metlife study of lesbian, gay, bisexual, and transgender baby boomers*. Westport, CT: MetLife Mature Market Institute. Retrieved from http://sageusa.org/resources/publications.dfm?ID=23

Meyer, I. H. (1995). Minority stress and mental health in gay men. *Journal of Health and Social Behavior*, *36*(1), 38–56.

Meyer, I. H. (2003). Prejudice, social stress, and mental health in lesbian, gay, and bisexual populations: Conceptual issues and research evidence. *Psychological Bulletin, 129*(5), 674–697.

Meyer, I. H., Dietrich, J., & Schwartz, S. (2008). Lifetime prevalence of mental disorders and suicide attempts in diverse lesbian, gay, and bisexual populations. *American Journal of Public Health, 98*, 1004–1006.

Murphy, Y., Hunt, V., Zajicek, A. M., Norris, A. N., & Hamilton, L. (2009). *Incorporating intersectionality in social work practice, research, policy, and education*. Washington, DC: NASW Press.

Nyitray, A., Corran, R., Altman, K., Chikani, V., & Negron, E. V. (2006). *Tobacco use and interventions among Arizona lesbian, gay, bisexual and transgender people*. Phoenix, AZ: Arizona Department of Health Services. Retrieved from http://www.lgbttobacco.org/files/Arizona_smoking_lgbt_report.pdf

Schope, R. D. (2005). Who's afraid of growing old? Gay and lesbian perceptions of aging. *Journal of Gerontological Social Work, 45*(4), 23–39.

Silverstein, C. (2009). The implications of removing homosexuality from the DSM as a mental disorder. *Archives of Sexual Behavior, 38*, 161–163.

Substance Abuse and Mental Health Services Administration. (2012). *Top Health Issues for LGBT Populations Information and Resource Kit*. HHS Publication No. (SMA) 12–4684. Rockville, MD: Substance Abuse and Mental Health Services Administration, 2012.

Travis, L. A., & Kimmel, D. C. (2014). Lesbian, gay, bisexual, and transgender ageing: Considerations for interventions. In N. A. Pachana & K. Laidlaw (Eds.), *Oxford handbook of clinical geropsychology* [Kindle version]. Oxford, UK: Oxford University Press.

Van Den Bergh, N., & Crisp, C. (2004). Defining culturally competent practice with sexual minorities: Implications for social work education and practice. *Journal of Social Work Education, 40*(2), 221–238.

Wallace, S. P., Cochran, S. D., Durazo, E. M., & Ford, C. L. (2011). The health of aging lesbian, gay and bisexual adults in California. *Policy Brief (UCLA Center for Health Policy Research)*, (0), 1–8.

Wight, R. G., LeBlanc, A. J., deVries, B., & Detels, R. (2012). Stress and mental health among midlife and older gay-identified men. *American Journal of Public Health, 102*(3), 503–510.

Wilson, B. D., & Miller, R. L. (2002). Strategies for managing heterosexism used among African American gay and bisexual men. *Journal of Black Psychology, 28*, 371–391.

Wilson, P. A. (2008). A dynamic-ecological model of identity formation and conflict among bisexually-behaving African-American men. *Archives of Sexual Behavior, 37*, 794–809.

Wilson, P. A., Valera, P., Ventuneac, A., Balan, I., Rowe, M., & Carballo-Dieguez, A. (2009). Race-based sexual stereotyping and sexual partnering among men who use the internet to identify other men for bareback sex. *Journal of Sex Research, 46*, 399–413.

Witten, T. M., & Eyler, A. E. (2012). *Gay, lesbian, bisexual, and transgender aging: Challenges in research, practice, and policy.* Baltimore: Johns Hopkins University Press.

Witten, T. M. (2014). It's not all darkness: Robustness, resilience, and successful transgender aging. *LGBT Health, 1*(1), 24–33.

World Health Organization. (2014). *Mental health: Strengthening our response.* Retrieved from http://www.who.int/mediacentre/factsheets/fs220/en

Wright, R., Owen, G., & Catalan, J. (2012). I'm older than I ever thought I would be: The lived experiences of ageing in HIV-positive gay men. In R. Ward, I. Rivers, & M. Sutherland (Eds.), *Lesbian, gay, bisexual and transgender ageing: Biographical approaches for inclusive care and support* (pp. 85–101). London, United Kingdom: Jessica Kingsley Publishers.

CHAPTER 6

Caregiving in the LGBT Community

Kristina M. Hash and Mariann Mankowski

ABSTRACT

Caregiving is a challenging yet rewarding life role that many individuals are called to fulfill for friends and family members. Research on caregiving for older adults has been growing rapidly in the past 30 years, identifying the many strains involved in as well as the positive outcomes of providing care. Only recently have studies in this area shed light on the experiences of sexual and gender minority caregivers and receivers. This body of research has illuminated the common challenges that face these individuals but also the unique stressors that they experience given their status. This chapter discusses the caregiving role in general as well as examines research specific to older lesbian, gay, bisexual, and transgender caregivers. The related topic of loss and bereavement as well as best practices and future directions with this population are also addressed.

BACKGROUND AND KEY CONCEPTS

Caregiving is the act and role of providing assistance to another individual and can be either formal or informal in nature. Formal caregivers include paid professionals such as home health aides, visiting nurses, and agency or organization volunteers who are unrelated or previously unknown to the care recipient.

http://dx.doi.org/10.1891/0198-8794.37.77

Informal caregivers are often parents, spouses, partners, family, and friends who provide care to individuals who are ill, disabled, or cannot perform activities of daily living. Caregiving for older loved ones has gained increasing attention in the gerontological literature over the past 30 years. The resulting studies have shown the caregiving role to be one that often produces negative outcomes for caregivers. The majority of caregiving tasks are often assumed by one person, called the primary caregiver, and this individual may experience the most negative outcomes. Most notably, strains related to finances, relationships, employment, and physical and mental health have been determined as outcomes of the caregiving role (George & Gwyther, 1986; Pinquart & Sorensen, 2003; Scharlach, Sobel, & Roberts, 1991; Schulz & Beach, 1999). These outcomes have been labeled stress, strain, and burden and instruments have been developed to measure these constructs and models have been created to understand these concepts and experiences (Pearlin, Mullen, Semple, & Skaff, 1990; Robinson, 1983; Vitaliano, Russo, Young, Becker, & Maiuro, 1991; Zarit, Reever, & Back-Peterson, 1980). The caregiving experience, however, has also been found to have positive impacts on the lives of caregivers such as being able to show love and commitment to a loved one, providing meaning to one's life, maintaining cultural expectations and responsivity for aging members, and avoiding the institutionalization of the care receiver (Cohen, Gold, Shulman, & Zucchero, 1994; Farran, Miller, Kaufman, Donner, & Fogg, 1999; Tarlow et al., 2004).

The majority of subjects in these caregiving studies have been or can be assumed to have been White, middle class, heterosexual individuals providing care for parents or parents-in-law or heterosexual spouses. Aside from the studies that examined caregiving for men with HIV/AIDS, the experiences of lesbian, gay, bisexual, and transgender (LGBT) caregivers has gone largely overlooked in the literature in this area. It is for certain, however, that gay male, lesbian, bisexual, and transgender persons have been and are involved in providing care to partners, spouses, and other loved ones. The literature in this area has shown that LGBT caregivers experience the same strains and positive outcomes as those in the general caregiving studies but must deal with additional strains related to their sexual orientation and gender identity (Brotman et al., 2007; Grossman, D'Augelli, & Dragowski, 2005; Hash, 2006; Metlife Mature Market Institute, 2010; Muraco & Fredriksen-Goldsen, 2014). This chapter examines the general caregiving literature as well as caregiving as it relates to older LGBT adults. As caregiving may end as the result of a death of a care receiver, the related topic of loss and bereavement is also discussed. The chapter concludes with a discussion of best practices and future directions with LGBT caregivers.

CURRENT RESEARCH ON LGBT CAREGIVING

The research related to the experience of caregiving and care receiving among aging LGBT individuals is distinct from the studies focusing on caregiving in the general population. The review below will detail what is currently known about caregiving and care receiving for this population and the challenges and benefits often experienced.

FAMILY OF CHOICE AND FAMILY OF ORIGIN

The literature on caregiving among aging LGBT adults identifies two different structures of informal care related to family life. These structures involve caring either by family of origin or by "families of choice" (Hostetler, 2004; MetLife, 2010). The family of origin typically consists of biologically connected individuals ("kin") either by birth or marriage and usually encompasses parents, siblings, children, former husbands and wives, and extended family members (Cruz, 2003; MetLife, 2010). Traditionally, these family members have been seen by the legal system as legitimate providers of care and care information. Families of choice involve same-sex partners, friends, and others who have been supportive of an individual's sexual orientation, gender identity, and relationships. A family of choice can also include blood relatives (Smith & Rapkin, 1996). The caregiving literature has examined the LGBT experience from both directions, that is, LGBT individuals as caregivers for family "kin" members, and family "kin" members providing care for LGB adults as care receivers (Muraco & Fredriksen-Goldsen, 2014).

Research on elder caregiving has shown the importance of social support in buffering the negative effects of the experience (Chappell & Funk, 2011; Haley, Levine, Brown, & Bartolucci, 1987; Spaid & Barusch, 1991). For aging LGBT caregivers and recipients this is vital given their life long experience of discrimination, oppression, and stigmatization (Herek, 1998). An important support systems for LGBT individuals are "families of choice," which frequently consists of same-sex partners, friends within the LGBT community, and an array of other relationally connected persons who are not "kin." Social support among aging LGBT individuals frequently involves members from families of origin and families of choice; the majority of social support comes from families of choice.

LGBT Individuals as Care Receivers

Family life is a dynamic and complex experience. Being the LGBT care recipient of support provided by family members (either family of origin or family of choice) offers both positive and negative experiences. On the one hand, LGB individuals are similar to all care recipients in that they appreciate the love, support, and assistance they receive from their family members. Similarly, they also report on the guilt, concern, and challenges they experience upon losing their independence and need for assistance (Muraco & Fredriksen-Goldsen, 2014). Yet, LGB caregivers and recipients also describe additional burdens and challenges because of their LGB status. For example, LGB caregivers report conflicts and challenges to their legitimacy in providing care from either family of origin members or institutions (Coon, Thompson, Steffen, Soccoro, & Gallagher-Thompson, 2003). Due to institutional requirements and privacy laws, health providers are permitted to share medical/health information with "next of kin" and often this does not include LGBT family of choice members (Mayer, Bradford, Makadon, Stall, Goldhammer, & Landers, 2008). Conflicts regarding the care recipient's sexual orientation or life style may have deep-seated roots among family of origin members creating barriers to caregiving, especially when given by nonkin family members. Witten (2009) reported that a lack of support from kinship families was due to historic estrangement, which prevented adequate care provision for LGBT care receivers. Family of choice networks assumed the largest majority of caregiving for older LGBT adults, and LGBT older adults would first turn to their partners and then friends before turning to other family members (Cahill, South, & Spade, 2000; de Vries, 2011).

LGBT INDIVIDUALS AS CAREGIVERS

LGBT caregivers to family of origin members have identified both the rewarding and challenging experiences of caring for "kin." Many caregivers report the value in caregiving as well as the responsibility they assume by caring for kin, in particular the pleasure they receive providing care for their family member (Brotman et al., 2007; Muraco & Fredriksen-Goldsen, 2014) and fulfilling cultural expectations to provide care for aging family members (Dilworth-Anderson, Brummett, Goodwin, Williams, Williams, & Siegler, 2005). LGBT family members who provide care for kin also report the burden and strain of family caregiving. They report the "double duty" they are oftentimes expected to maintain by caregiving for their family member and continuing with the responsibilities of their daily lives such as employment and home life. Shippy (2007) examined the support and resources among LGB persons and found almost half of their study subjects (N = 155) were caregivers to members of both their biological and choice families. Frequently, LGB adults report there is an assumption among their heterosexual family members that they do not experience burden because their lifestyle is not defined in terms of a traditional lifestyle. This can result in conflicts among siblings, children, parents, extended family members, and the care recipient (Hash, 2006).

STRAINS AND BENEFITS INVOLVED IN LGBT CAREGIVING

Recent literature on LGB caregiving also identified the strains and benefits of caregiving and care receiving (Cantor, Brennan, & Shippy, 2004; Croghan, Moone, & Olson, 2012; Hash, 2006; Hash & Netting, 2009; Muraco & Fredriksen-Goldsen, 2014). Strain may be experienced by the caregiver as a result of the stress of providing care for biological or choice family members (Croghan, Moone, & Olson, 2012). Significant strain can occur when the caregiver is employed outside the home, when the caregiver is not "out" at work or in their community, or when the family of origin is conflicted by the sexual orientation of their LGBT family member (Grossman et al., 2005; Hash, 2006). Furthermore, providing care can cause physical strain that can have negative health implications for both the caregiver and care receiver (Spillman & Long, 2009; Stull, Kosloski, & Kercher, 1994). The care receiver can also experience strain related to feelings associated with not wanting to be a burden and embarrassment over needing assistance (Muraco & Fredriksen-Goldsen, 2014).

Isolation can be a strain for aging LGBT adults, regardless of whether they are involved in caregiving. In fact, older LGBT adults are at greater risk for isolation than their non-LGBT peers, and being alone with no one to care for them is a significant fear for many members of this population (Brennan-Ing et al., 2014; Fredriksen-Goldsen et al., 2011; Hash, 2006; Shippy, 2007). Fredriksen-Goldsen et al.'s (2011) study of over 2,500 older LGBT adults found that transgender adults and bisexual men experienced the highest levels of isolation (with over 60% reporting this problem), while gay men, lesbians, and bisexual women reported slightly less isolation. In terms of isolation, specific risk factors for this population include the fact that that older LGBT adults are less likely to be partnered or married, less likely to have children, and more likely to live alone and be estranged from their families of origin than their non-LGBT peers. This experience of isolation can compound the other strains involved in caregiving.

Accessing formal support services for LGBT caregivers and receivers can also serve as significant stressors. In general, formal care, such as supports provided by agencies, health care centers, and community programs, is utilized as a last resort by many aging LGBT adults. Accessing formal care is viewed with trepidation by LGBT adults for a number of reasons. Primary concerns regarding the utilization of formal care include fears of discrimination, denial of services because of sexual and gender minority status, and feelings of not being welcome (Brotman et al., 2007; Croghan, Moone, & Olsen, 2012; Hash, 2006; Hughes, 2009; Knochel, Croghan, Moone, & Quam, 2012). Formal care provided by institutions is the subject of even greater distress for LGBT caregivers and receivers. Although only 5% of all aging adults are housed in skilled nursing facilities, the majority of aging adults report fear of placement in these facilities as their primary concern (Hillier & Barrow, 2010). A national survey by Area Agencies on Aging (AAA) report these concerns may be realistic, as less than 13% of AAA conducted outreach to older LGBT adults and a 7-year review of conference sessions reported a small number (8 out of 1,136) targeted services toward older LGBT adults or trained their staff on LGBT issues (Knochel, Croghan, Moone, & Quam, 2012).

Caregiving and receiving among this population has also been found to have many benefits. Most often older LGBT adults describe their caregiving and care receiving from a relational context with caregiving as experienced interpersonally as altruistic feelings of "giving back" or "paying it forward," and many caregivers feel they receive more than they give when providing care (Brotman et al., 2007; Muraco & Fredriksen-Goldsen, 2014). Personal growth, feeling good about oneself, experiencing greater closeness and commitment, and fulfilling an obligation to a loved one can also serve as benefits to providing care (Hash, 2006). Similarly, care recipients experience the benefit of being protected and or cared for, which for some, is affirming given a lifetime of discrimination and marginalization. The caregiving dyadic exchange is described as an active participation between both parties (Lyons et al., 2002).

BEREAVEMENT IN THE LGBT COMMUNITY

The topic of bereavement is important to discuss, as the caregiving experience will often lead to the loss of a care receiver. As with caregiving, the research in the area of bereavement among LGBT individuals has identified unique features for this population. Unfortunately, this research is quite limited and the experiences of transgender elders are not represented. For same-sex couples, not having fully disclosed the nature of the partner relationship can prove difficult in the face of loss and bereavement. "Disenfranchised grief" (Doka 1989, 2002) can accurately describe this type of loss that involves a loss that one is not able to publically acknowledge or mourn. It is also one that may not be accepted or identified as legitimate by family, friends, coworkers, or even policies. Studies of older same-sex partner bereavement have shown that these widows/widowers may have difficulty accessing formal and informal supports (such as grief support groups) because of the fear of being open about the nature of their same-sex relationship. Individuals who lose a same-sex partner may be at particular risk for isolation, although "family of choice" can provide a great deal of support during bereavement (Almack, Seymour, & Bellamy, 2010; Fenge, 2014; Hash, 2006).

For LGBT older adults who are now legally married to partners of the same gender, the recent legalization of marriage for same-sex couples in the United States should provide protections for individuals who provide care for and then lose a spouse. Qualifying for survivor benefits through Social Security and the Veterans Administration and the removal of inheritance penalties are two major policy changes that resulted from marriage legalization and have great potential to improve the lives of LGBT widows and widowers.

BEST PRACTICES AND FUTURE DIRECTIONS

Caregiving for older loved ones involves strain and negative outcomes as well as positive impacts for individuals, regardless of sexual orientation or gender identity. LGBT caregivers experience added strain due to their identities and relationships and the policies and societal attitudes that surround them. By the year 2030, the number of aging sexual and gender minority adults is expected to reach approximately 4 million (Fredriksen-Goldsen et al., 2011). From this projection, it can be assumed that in the future there will be an increased need for caregiving among this population.

Many program models have been developed to assist caregivers and receivers, and these models can benefit all. Best practices and interventions developed for general caregiving populations, such as Resources for Enhancing Alzheimer's Caregiver Health (REACH II) program and those funded by National Family Caregiver Support Program (Older Americans Act Title IIIE), can benefit LGBT caregiving situations as well. To reach the most vulnerable aging care recipients and their caregivers requires caregiver programs and resources to consider the unique needs and fears of older LGBT adults in their service delivery. For example, coordinated care is needed with the awareness that many older LGBT adults may not be "out" to informal or formal support persons, as they have lived the majority of their lives in times when their identities and LGBT relationships were not supported and were often criminalized and marginalized. It is equally important that community agencies understand the special health care needs of this population as well as the mental health conditions for which they may be at risk. In addition, coordinating care that recognizes some older LGBT individuals and couples have built strong support networks to protect against societal and familial marginalization is essential. This includes calling upon "families of choice" members to provide a variety of assistance (Weston, 1991).

With regard to service provision for older LGBT caregivers and care receivers, Services and Advocacy for GLBT Elders (SAGE; www.sageusa.org) has operated the Partners in Caring Program in New York City since 2004 and the Caring and Preparing program since 2009. Several SAGE-affiliated organizations have also opened throughout the United States. SAGE and the National Resource Center on LGBT Aging also launched an online LGBT Caregiver Resource Center. Beyond formal service and health organizations, specialized support communities have been developed by and for older LGBT adults and may be even more prevalent in the future. Retirement communities are being developed for LGBT aging adults across the United States (i.e., Palms of Manasota in Florida). Other older LGBT adults choose to form communities of friends and family when they retire to provide a caring community (Hash & Netting, 2009).

Policies have also been implemented to ease the burden of the caregiving experience for older LGBT adults. Even prior to the legalization of same-sex marriage, hospital visitation rights were granted to same-sex couples starting in 2011, and the federal Family Medical Leave Act of 1993 now protects same-sex couples. The Lifespan Respite Care Act of 2006 provides grants to states to provide programming to give respite to caregivers, including LGBT caregivers. In the majority of states, Medicaid also covers some respite services for caregivers. In the 2000 reauthorization of the Older Americans Act, the National Family Caregiver Support Program was established and provides nationwide information and referral to family caregivers. Federal tax deductions are also allowed for some caregiving-related expenses (Lipson, 2015). As previously mentioned, many policies related to bereavement now benefit same-sex couples. Unfortunately, policies benefitting transgender persons have not reached the same level of progress, particularly those related to health care.

In terms of research in this area, a great deal has been learned about the strains and benefits of caregiving for older adults in a body of literature that has been accumulating over the past three decades. The LGBT caregiving literature, however, is still in its infancy and its unique features still require additional inquiry and validation. As this knowledge grows, it can be disseminated to organizations, professionals, and educators to ensure sensitive and appropriate health and social services for older gay, lesbian, bisexual, and transgender caregivers and receivers.

REFERENCES

Almack, K., Seymour, J., & Bellamy, G. (2010). Exploring the impact of sexual orientation on experiences and concerns about end of life care and on bereavement for lesbian, gay and bisexual elders. *Sociology, 44*(5), 908–924.

Brennan-Ing, M., Seidel, L., Larson, B., & Karpiak, S. E. (2014). Social care networks and older LGBT adults: Challenges for the future. *Journal of Homosexuality, 61*, 21–52.

Brotman, S., Ryan, B., Collins, S., Chamberland, L., Cormier, R., Julien, D., et al. (2007). Coming out to care: Caregivers of gay and lesbian seniors in Canada. *Gerontologist, 47*(4), 490–503.

Cahill, S., South, K., & Spade, J. (2000). *Outing age: Public policy issues affecting gay, lesbian, bisexual, and transgender elders.* Washington, DC: National Gay and Lesbian Task Force.

Cantor, M. H., Brennan, M., & Shippy, R. A. (2004). *Caregiving among older lesbian, gay, bisexual and transgender New Yorkers*. New York, NY: Policy Institute of the National Gay and Lesbian Task Force.

Chappell, N. L., & Funk, L. M. (2011). Social support, caregiving, and aging. *Canadian Journal on Aging, 30*(3), 355–370.

Cohen, C. A., Gold, D. P., Shulman, K. I., & Zucchero, D. A. (1994). Positive aspects in caregiving: An overlooked variable in research. *Canadian Journal on Aging 13,* 378–391.

Cohen, H. L., & Murray, Y. (2006). Older lesbian and gay caregivers: Caring for families of choice and caring for families of origin. *Journal of Human Behavior in the Social Environment, 14*(1/2), 275–298

Coon, D. W. (2005). Exploring interventions for LGBT caregivers: Issues and examples. *Journal of Gay and Lesbian Social Services, 18*(3/4), 109–128.

Coon, D. W., Thompson, L., Steffen, A., Soccoro, K., & Gallagher-Thompson, D. (2003). Anger and depression management: Psychoeducational skill training interventions for women caregivers of a relative with dementia. *Gerontologist, 43*, 678–689.

Croghan, C., Moone, R., & Olson, A. (2012). *Twin Cities LGBT aging needs assessment survey*. Minneapolis, MN: Greater Twin Cities United Way and PFund Foundation.

Cruz, J. (2003). *Sociological analysis of aging: The gay male perspective*. Binghamton, NY: Harrington Park Press.

de Vries, B. (2011). LGBT aging: Research and policy directions. *Public Policy and Aging Report, 21*(3), 34–35.

Dilworth-Anderson, P., Brummett, B. H., Goodwin, P., Williams, S. W., Williams, R. B., & Siegler, I. C. (2005). Effect of race on cultural justification for caregiving. *Journal of Gerontology, 60*(5), 257–262.

Doka, K. (1989). *Disenfranchised grief: Recognizing hidden sorrow*. New York, NY: Lexington Books.

Doka, K. (2002). *Disenfranchised grief: New directions, challenges and strategies for practice*. Champaign, IL: Research Press.

Farran, C., Miller, B., Kaufman, J., Donner, E., & Fogg, L. (1999). Finding meaning through caregiving: Development of an instrument for family caregivers of persons with Alzheimer's Disease. *Journal of Clinical Psychology, 9*, 1107–1125.

Fenge, L. (2014). Developing understanding of same-sex partner bereavement for older lesbian and gay people: Implications for social work practice. *Journal of Gerontological Social Work, 57*(2–4), 288–304.

Fredriksen-Goldsen, K. I., Kim, H. J., Emlet, C. A., Muraco, A., Erosheva, E. A., Hoy-Ellis, C. P., et al. (2011). *The aging and health report: Disparities and resilience among lesbian, gay, bisexual, and transgender older adults*. Seattle, WA: Institute for Multigenerational Health.

George, L. K., & Gwyther, L. P. (1986). Caregiver well-being: A multidimensional examination of family caregivers of demented adults. *The Gerontologist, 26*(3), 253–259.

Grossman, A. H., D'Augelli, A. R., & Dragowski, E. A. (2005). Caregiving and care receiving among older lesbian, gay, and bisexual adults. *Journal of Gay and Lesbian Social Services, 18*(3/4), 15–38.

Haley, W. E., Levine, E. G., Brown, S. L., & Bartolucci, A. A. (1987). Stress, appraisal, coping, and social support as predictors of adaptational outcome among dementia caregivers. *Psychology and Aging, 2*(4), 323–330.

Hash, K. M. (2006). Caregiving and post-caregiving experiences of midlife and older gay men and lesbians. *Journal of Gerontological Social Work, 47*(3/4), 121–138.

Hash, K. M. & Netting, F. E. (2009). It takes a community: Older lesbians meeting social and care needs. *Journal of Gay and Lesbian Social Services, 21*, 326–342.

Herek, G. (1998). *Stigma and sexual orientation: Understanding prejudice against lesbians, gay men and bisexuals*. Thousand Oaks, CA: Sage.

Hillier, S. & Barrow, G. (2010). *Aging, individual and society* (9th ed.). Belmont, CA: Wadsworth.

Hostetler, A. (2004). Old, gay, and alone? The ecology of well-being among middle-aged and older single gay men. In G. Herdt & B. de Vries (Eds.), *Gay and lesbian aging: Research and future directions* (pp. 143–176). New York, NY: Springer Publishing.

Hughes, M. (2009). Lesbian and gay people's concerns about ageing and accessing services. *Australian Social Work, 62*, 186–201.

Knochel, K. A., Coghan, C. F., Moone, R., & Quam, J. (2012). Training, geography and provision of aging services to lesbian, gay, bisexual, and transgender older adults. *Journal of Gerontological Social Work, 55*, 426–443.

Lipson, D. (2015). *Family caregiving: 20 years of public policy.* Retrieved from https://www.mathematica-mpr.com/our-publications-and-findings/publications/family-caregiving-20-years-of-federal-policy

Lyons, K. S., Zarit, S. H., Sayer, A. G., & Whitlatch, C. J. (2002). Caregiving as a dyadic process: Perspectives from caregiver and receiver. *Journals of Gerontology Series B, 57B*, 195–204.

Mayer, K. H., Bradford, J. B., Makadon, H. J., Stall, R., Goldhammer, H., & Landers, S. (2008). Sexual and gender minority health: What we know and what needs to be done. *American Journal of Public Health, 98*(6), 989–995.

Metlife Mature Market Institute. (2010). *Still out, still aging: The Metlife study of lesbian gay, bisexual, and transgendered baby boomers*. Westport, CT: Metlife.

Muraco, A., & Fredriksen-Goldsen, K. I. (2014). The highs and lows of caregiving for chronically Ill lesbian, gay, and bisexual elders. *Journal of Gerontological Social Work, 57*(2–4), 251–272.

Pearlin, L. I., Mullan, J. T., Semple, S. J., & Skaff, M. M. (1990). Caregiving and the stress process: An overview of concepts and their measures. *The Gerontologist, 30*(5), 583–594.

Pinquart, M., & Sörensen, S. (2003). Differences between caregivers and noncaregivers in psychological health and physical health: a meta-analysis. *Psychology and Aging, 18*(2), 250.

Robinson, B. C. (1983). Validation of a caregiver strain index. *Journal of Gerontology, 38*(3), 344–348.

Scharlach, A. E., Sobel, E. L., & Roberts, R. E. (1991). Employment and caregiver strain: An integrative model. *The Gerontologist, 31*(6), 778–787.

Schulz, R., & Beach, S. R. (1999). Caregiving as a risk factor for mortality: The Caregiver Health Effects Study. *JAMA, 282*(23), 2215–2219.

Shippy, R. A. (2007). We cannot go it alone: The impact of informal support and stressors in older gay, lesbian, and bisexual caregivers. *Journal of Gay and Lesbian Social Services, 18*(3/4), 39–51.

Smith, M. Y., & Rapkin, B. D. (1996). Social support and barriers to family involvement in caregiving_for persons with AIDS: Implications for patient education. *Patient Education and Counseling, 27*(1), 85–94.

Spaid, W. M., & Barusch, A. S. (1991). Social support and caregiver strain: types and sources of social contacts of elderly caregivers. *Journal of Gerontological Social Work, 18*(1–2), 151–161.

Spillman, B. & Long, S. (2009). Does high caregiver stress predict nursing home entry? *Inquiry, 46*, 140–161.

Stull, D. E., Kosloski, K., & Kercher, K. (1994). Caregiver burden and generic well-being: opposite sides of the same coin? *Gerontologist, 34*(1), 88–94.

Tarlow, B. J., Wisniewski, S. R., Belle, S. H., Rubert, M., Ory, M. G., & Gallagher-Thompson, D. (2004). Positive aspects of caregiving: Contributions of the REACH project to the development of new measures for Alzheimer's caregiving. *Research on Aging, 26*(4), 429–453.

Vitaliano, P. P., Russo, J., Young, H. M., Becker, J., & Maiuro, R. D. (1991). The screen for caregiver burden. *The Gerontologist, 31*(1), 76–83.

Weston, K. (1991). *Families we choose: Lesbians, gays, kinship*. New York, NY: Columbia University Press.

Witten, T. M. (2009). Graceful exits: Intersection of aging, transgender identities, and the family/community. *Journal of GLBT Family Studies, 5*(1/2), 35–61.

Zarit, S. H., Reever, K. E., & Back-Peterson, J. (1980). Relatives of the impaired elderly: Correlates of feelings of burden. *The Gerontologist, 20*, 649–655.

CHAPTER 7

Families and Support Systems of LGBT Elders

Nancy A. Orel

ABSTRACT

Families and social support systems have been found to be instrumental for the physical and psychological well-being of older adults. However, the majority of research on families has assumed that all members within a family are heterosexual. This chapter discusses families and social support systems for lesbian, gay, bisexual, and transgender (LGBT) older adults. The chapter initially provides an overview of the research on social networks and social support systems of the general older adult population. The discussion on LGBT older adults' families and social support systems highlights families of choice, LGBT communities, and the impact of disclosing one's sexual orientation on social network relationships. The chapter concludes with recommendations for future research and best practices that focus on addressing the unique needs and concerns of LGBT elders.

INTRODUCTION

Within gerontological research, family has been identified as the dominant social group in the lives of older individuals. Peter Townsend (1957) in his book *The Family Life of Old People*, concluded that:

> if many of the processes and problems of ageing are to be understood, old people must be studied as members of families (which usually means extended

http://dx.doi.org/10.1891/0198-8794.37.89

> families of three generations); and if this is true, those concerned with health and social administration must, at every stage, treat old people as an inseparable part of a family group, which is more than just a residential unit. They are not simply individuals, let alone 'cases' occupying beds or chairs. They are members of families and whether or not they are treated as such largely determines their security, their health, and their happiness. (p. 19)

Townsend was one of the first researchers to argue that families and social support systems are instrumental for the physical and psychological well-being of older adults. However, Townsend did not address the fact that modifications were necessary in his view of aging family members when one considers the diversity that exists to define families. From a historical perspective, the nuclear family and its older family members were seen as being instrumental for the survival of the society, and there was close geographical proximity between all members of the family. However, by the 1960s, older adults were becoming more independent and the geographical distance between relatives was increasing; thus social mobility and geographical mobility influenced the development of a new type of family where reciprocity between the generations decreased.

Most importantly, Townsend did not address the fact that modifications were necessary in his view of aging family members if one is considering families and social support systems of lesbian, gay, bisexual, and transgender (LGBT) older adults. Specifically, many LGBT elders have been estranged from their families of origin, and instead the importance of families of choice (Weston, 1997) must be recognized and honored when considering the social networks of LGBT older adults. Families of choice or chosen families is a term used to describe kin networks that LGBT individuals developed out of necessity when they were estranged from their biological families. Families of choice usually include partners, friends, coworkers, neighbors, and ex-partners and these individuals provide the emotional and instrumental support that would be expected from one's family of origin (de Vries & Megathlin, 2009). According to Kimmel, Rose, Orel, and Greene (2005), "LGBT individuals have a variety of family life cycle patterns and may be in different places in their cycle than their heterosexual peers" (p. 7). Townsend's early research reflected the early social and cultural bias of giving too much emphasis on sociability and social support inside people's homes—through their families of origin—and not enough on friendships and/or families of choice that can replicate families of origin within a variety of settings.

Erosheva, Kim, Emlet, and Fredriksen-Goldsen (2015) in their examination of social networks of LGBT older adults clearly indicated that the research on the physical and psychological benefits of families and social support systems for LGBT individuals is limited, with research on LGBT older adults even more limited. However, research has shown that there are both physical and psychological benefits of families and social support systems for the general older adult population. Older adults who are "embedded in resource-rich social networks experience better well-being, better mental health, and other health benefits compared to those in resource-poor networks" (Erosheva et al., 2015, p. 2).

This chapter discusses families and social support systems of LGBT older adults and highlights the physical and psychological benefits of these familial and social support systems for LGBT older adults. Prior to beginning this discussion, it is important to provide an overview of the research on social networks among the general older adult population. The discussion of families and social support systems of LGBT older adults includes a review on families of origin, families of choice, and LGBT communities. Throughout the discussion on families and social support systems of LGBT older adults, an exploration of the ways in which disclosing one's sexual orientation affects social network relationships, experiences, and outcomes is emphasized. When discussing families and social support systems of LGBT older adults, it is imperative that the issue of managing disclosure is highlighted.

BACKGROUND, KEY CONCEPTS, AND CURRENT RESEARCH SOCIAL NETWORKS OF THE GENERAL OLDER ADULT POPULATION

Social networks are "the collection of interpersonal and communal bonds that people have throughout their lives to establish social relations that satisfy certain needs, and maintain their well-being" (Doubova, Perez Cuevas, Espinosa-Alcron, & Flores-Hernadez, 2010, p. 1). Generally, social networks include relationships with family, friends, neighbors, acquaintances, colleagues, coworkers, members of the community, and members of online networking sites (Erosheva et al., 2015). Litwin and Landau (2000) indicate that network types are characterized by criteria such as "size, composition, percentage of intimate ties, frequency of contact, duration of ties, and geographic proximity" (p. 217). Networks types provide varying levels of social support and have varying effects on their members.

Gerontological research has examined the social networks of older adults. Important determinants of social networks among the general older adult population include marital status, family relations, religious activities, and membership in organizations (Fiori, Smith, & Antonucci, 2007; Gray, 2009; Litwin & Shiovitz-Ezra, 2011). The research on the social networks of older adults indicates that individuals who are currently in marital relationships have larger social networks (Cicirelli, 2010; Hurlbert & Acock, 1990; McLaughlin, Vagenas, Pachana, Begum, & Dobson, 2010), and older adults with children have larger social networks (Conway, Magai, Jones, Fiori, & Gillespie, 2013). Glass and Balfour (2003) reported that older persons, in comparison to younger populations, consider community organizations (e.g., senior centers) and community entities (neighborhoods) to be important aspects of their social networks.

The types and size of social networks that older individuals create can vary based on cultural attributes such as race, gender, nationality, and socioeconomic status (Doubova et al., 2010; Fiori, Smith, & Antonucci, 2007; Litwin & Schiovitz-Ezra, 2011). Previous research has indicated that older women have larger social networks than men (Cicirelli, 2010) and that older adults with higher socioeconomic statuses tend to have larger and more diverse social networks (Ajrouch, Blandon, & Antonucci, 2005). Cornwell, Laumann, and Schumm (2008) reported that African American and Hispanic older adults generally have smaller social networks than Whites, and the size of social networks diminishes with age. Some research indicates that older adults who have retired have larger social networks (Cornwell et al., 2008). However, if these same older adults are experiencing chronic illness, then their social networks tend to decrease in size, which in turn reduces available social supports (McLaughlin et al., 2010).

SOCIAL SUPPORT SYSTEMS OF THE GENERAL OLDER ADULT POPULATION

A distinction should be made between the concepts of social networks and social support. Social networks entail a set of social bonds among an identified group of people, characterized by the social behaviors of the people involved. Social support is an interactive process whereby emotional, instrumental, informational (e.g., advice), or tangible (e.g., financial) assistance is obtained from one's social network (Berkman & Glass, 2000). Social support also includes companionship or the sense of belongingness. Social support is usually measured by the amount of assistance received. However, an individual's *perception* of assistance available from pets, family, friends, neighbors, coworkers, organizations, government, and so on can also be a measure of social support.

Social support has been identified as being instrumental for the physical and psychological well-being of individuals, essential for maintaining physical and psychological health, and may enhance one's resilience to stress (Ozbay et al., 2007). Social support has also been found to have a significant impact on both mortality and morbidity; the lack of social support has been found to be detrimental to one's physical and emotional health and well-being (Ozbay et al., 2007).

Generally, research has indicated that older adults often have diminished social support, heightened levels of loneliness, and lower life satisfaction (Adams,

Sanders, & Auth, 2004). As individuals age, their social networks often decline in number, and these declines are often due to normative, age-related life events (Wrzus, Hanel, Wagner, & Neyer, 2013). Older adults face the loss of friends, family, or acquaintances to death, retirement, or relocation. The ability of older adults to establish new friendships may be hindered if they are experiencing physical health issues that reduce their mobility. However, some older adults with diminished capacity may move to assisted living facilities that often provide numerous opportunities to establish new friendships. Many older adults are discovering that the Internet (e.g., e-mail, Skype) allows them to maintain contacts that in the past were maintained through phone calls or handwritten letters or cards, reducing loneliness and improving quality of life (Cotton, Anderson, & McCullough, 2013).

Older adults are at risk for social isolation, often when they are no longer actively engaged within their broader communities (e.g., schools, work settings, community organizations, and places of worship) or engaged with their friends and families. The primary risk factor for this isolation among older adults is living alone. Other risk factors include physical and/or cognitive impairments, mobility difficulties, and low socioeconomic status. The consequences of social isolation include smaller social support networks, feelings of loneliness and depression, and deterioration of physical and mental health (Erosheva et al., 2015).

LGBT OLDER ADULTS' SOCIAL NETWORKS

LGBT older adults may be disproportionately more vulnerable to social isolation than heterosexual older adults because LGBT elders are twice as likely to live alone and be single, and three to four times less likely to have children (Erosheva et al., 2015). Additionally, some LGBT older adults may live within a geographical region that does not have adequate LGBT-friendly community and service support systems for older adults (Hasenbush, Flores, Kastanis, Sears, & Gates, 2014).

A growing body of evidence dispels the once held belief that all LGBT older adults are socially isolated (Wrzus et al., 2013). This research indicates that older gay men and lesbians may have sources of social networks and support including friends, partners, neighbors, as well as members of their "families of choice," biological families, and the LGBT community (Grossman, D'Augelli, & O'Connell, 2001; Orel, 2004). These various types of families and sources of social support are instrumental for the health and well-being of LGBT older adults.

Limited research exists on the social networks of LGBT older adults; however, two early studies indicated that gay men organize their social networks differently than heterosexual men (Nardi, 1999; Woolwine, 2000) and the differences were attributed to the stigmatized status that gay men have within society. More recently, Cook-Daniels (2015) found that transgender older adults, when compared to nontransgender older adults, have larger social networks. Fredrikson-Goldsen et al. (2013) further found that among LGB older adults, social network size and social support were protective factors. The existence of both social support and social networks decreased the likelihood of poor general health, disability, and depression. This same study indicated that the size of the social network tempered or attenuated the relationship between internalized stigma and poor general health in LGB older adults. Most significantly, current research suggests that the majority of lesbian and gay baby boomers have acceptance from their families of origin (Metlife, 2010).

SOCIAL SUPPORT FROM FAMILIES OF ORIGIN FOR LGBT OLDER ADULTS

Many LGBT older adults maintain strong ties with their families of origin while living openly as LGBT individuals (Connidis, 2010; Fullmer, 2006; Heaphy, 2009). Heaphy's (2009) research with 266 gay men and lesbian women over the age of 50 found that 67% of the participants reported that their "relationships with family members were important," they "were open about their sexuality and same-sex relationships to at least some relatives," and that "relationships with families of origin were, therefore, more important than is suggested by much of the existing literature" (Heaphy, 2009, p. 128). However, bisexual older adults reported less accepting families than their gay or lesbian counterparts (MetLife, 2010) and older transgender people reported complex family relationships (Witten & Eyler, 2012).

For the majority of individuals in the general population, families provide key sources of social, economic, educational, and emotional support throughout the life span (Demo, Allen, & Fine, 2000). Researchers have documented the importance of family relationships, especially for older adults who may require assistance and direct care from their families. Scherrer and Fedor (2015) provided an overview of the existing scholarship about LGBT older adults and their families of origin and identified key issues that LGBT older adults confront in their familial relationships. One of the key issues identified was the variety of LGBT older adults' definitions of family.

Fredriksen-Goldsen (2009) also highlighted the diversity of families among LGBT older adults. For example, LGBT older adults may belong to families that include LGBT parents and heterosexual children/grandchildren, LGBT couples with no children, and LGBT couples who have either formalized their relationships earlier through a civil union or more recently through legal same-sex marriage. LGBT persons actively participate in their roles as sons, daughters, sisters, brothers, nieces, nephews, uncles, and aunts. However, for some LGBT older adults, their life-course experiences included "choosing between living an authentic life as an LGBT person and maintaining ties with their families of origin" (Scherrer & Fedor, 2015, p. 178). Research suggests that families of origin that support and accept their LGBT family members promote a sense of belonging and support that is associated with feelings of well-being for LGBT family members (Orel, 2006).

In any discussion of families and support systems of LGBT elders, it is imperative to consider the social context LGBT older adults have experienced. Most, if not all, LGBT older adults lived in a social context that prevented them from disclosing their sexual orientation or gender identity from members of their family of origin. Many LGBT older adults lived a double life "in the closet" (Seidman, 2002) because homosexuality was viewed as immoral, deviant, and criminal. For example, LGBT elders who are currently aged 75 and older have witnessed the state department hearings and subsequent dismissal of employees based on allegations of homosexuality (1950); the inclusion of homosexuality as a psychopathological disorder in the *Diagnostic and Statistical Manual of Mental Disorders* (*DSM*; 1952); the Stonewall Riots (1969); the assassination of Harvey Milk, San Francisco's first openly gay elected city supervisor (1978); reported cases of "unexplained" deaths among gay males in San Francisco, referred to as "gay related infectious disease" (1981); the brutal murder of Matthew Shepard (1998); Reverend Jerry Falwell's suggestion that homosexuals were partly responsible for the September 11 terrorist attack on the World Trade Center (2001); and the Sixth U.S. Circuit Court of Appeals decision that upheld same-sex marriage bans in four Midwest states (2014). Although most LGBT older adults have also witnessed key positive historical events (e.g., removal of homosexuality as a disease category from the *DSM* [1973], the gay march on Washington DC [1987], creation of the national LGBT resource center [2010], the end of the ban of gays and lesbians serving in the military [2011], the Supreme Court ruling that same-sex couples can marry nationwide [2015]), there continues to be a lack of federal protection against anti-LGBT workplace discrimination.

Based on pervasive heterosexism and homophobia that all LGBT older adults have witnessed or personally experienced, many LGBT individuals remained closeted to friends, neighbors, coworkers, family members, and medical professionals. LGBT individuals faced countless situations where they had to make the conscious and deliberate decision to disclose or manage information about their sexual orientation. As such, the coming out process and/or managing disclosure has been a lifelong and difficult process for many LGBT older adults. Because the current LGBT older adult population personally experienced homophobic social conditions, they were (and continue to be) less likely than current cohorts of LGBT individuals to be open about their sexual orientation or gender identity within all social contexts (Morrow, 2006; Seidman, 2002), but especially within their families of origin (Heaphy, 2009; Witten, 2009). Although some social conditions have changed, some older LGBT individuals remain hesitant about disclosing their sexual orientation or gender identity to friends, colleagues, coworkers, and/or family members. A participant in a recent survey of LGBT older adults in Northeast Ohio reported that "the mental strength required to constantly remain closeted is often compared to the exertion needed to hold and keep a beach ball under water" (LGBT Community Center of Greater Cleveland, 2015, p. 26).

Coming out can have potentially negative physical, financial, legal, emotional, and social consequences, but coming out can also have psychological and social benefits. For example, disclosing one's homosexuality increases the likelihood of meeting similar others. However, all LGBT individuals must go through a thoughtful deliberation of both the potential positive and negative consequences of coming out, particularly to family members including children and grandchildren.

LGBT OLDER ADULTS AND THEIR ADULT CHILDREN AND GRANDCHILDREN

Few studies have explored LGBT older adults' relationships with their adult children. Connidis (2010) attributed this lack of research to a "reluctance to acknowledge the families of gay and lesbian individuals" (p. 143). Research on LGBT persons who are mothers and fathers has increased within the past decade, with research on lesbian mothers being the most common. The majority of this research has focused on gay and lesbian people who have biological or adoptive children from prior heterosexual relationships (Cronin, Ward, Pugh, & Price, 2011; Hunter, 2005; Tasker, 2013). Although accurate estimates of the number of lesbian and gay individuals who are parents are not available, Heaphy's (2009) research found that 42% of lesbians and 24% of gay men were parents.

Many LGBT parents elect never to disclose their sexual orientation to their children, while others may wait until later in life when their children are adults (Connidis, 2010; Hunter, 2005). Some research indicates that when children suspect their parents' sexual orientation, the coming out process can be indirect if these children share their suspicions with their parents and subsequently the parents confirm their children's assumptions about their sexual orientation (Hunter, 2005). Even less research has explored how adult children respond to the realization that a parent is LGBT. Witten and Eyler (2012) reported that adult children whose transgender parents disclose their gender identity may face unique challenges related to the use of new pronouns, preferred names, and the use of family names such as mom or dad.

The current cohort of LGBT older adults with adult children most likely had their children within the context of a previous non-LGBT relationship, and many of these LGBT older adults did not fully realize their sexual orientation or gender identity until later in life (Fullmer, 2006; Hunter, 2005), long after having given birth to children. Consequently, some LGBT older adults may now be both a parent and a grandparent faced with the decision to disclose their sexual orientation to adult children and/or grandchildren.

Historically, research on grandparenthood has assumed that grandparents were heterosexual. Accurate estimates of the current number of LGBT grandparents are not available, but it is estimated that 94% of older adults with children will become grandparents and 50% will become great grandparents (Smith & Drew, 2002). Applying these statistics to the estimated 3 million lesbian and gay parents, a conservative range of 1 to 2 million lesbians and gay men are grandparents (or will become grandparents). The number of same-sex parents is increasing (Goldberg, 2010) and as a result, greater numbers of LGBT individuals will experience grandparenthood than previous cohorts of LGBT individuals.

Research on LGBT grandparents is still limited despite the fact that research on LGBT parents has increased within the past decade (Goldberg, 2010). Research on LGBT grandparents has primarily focused on lesbian grandmothers and gay grandfathers. Relatively little scholarship on bisexual grandparents exists, and to date there is no research on transgender people as grandparents.

Orel (2004, 2006), Orel and Fruhauf (2006), and Fruhauf, Orel, and Jenkins (2009) explored the effects of sexual orientation on the grandparent–grandchild relationship using the life-course perspective. These authors indicated that the LGB grandparent–grandchild relationship is embedded within the context of the LGB grandparents' individual choices across the life span (e.g., decisions to disclose one's homosexuality), the structural contexts in which these decisions are made (e.g., level of homophobia within a culture), and the transitions that LGB grandparents experienced (e.g., previous heterosexual marriages and divorces; Orel & Fruhauf, 2015).

In this research, descriptions of LGB grandparents' relationships with their grandchildren were always placed within the context of their ongoing relationships with their adult children. This finding was similar to previous research on the grandparent–grandchild relationship with heterosexual grandparents where adult children are the intermediaries of the grandparent–grandchild relationship. Adult children facilitate or discourage relationships between grandparents and grandchildren. However, adult children as intermediaries is amplified for

LGB grandparents and this was most evident through the adult child's attitudes toward homosexuality. Adult children who were accepting of their parent's sexual orientation assisted in answering questions and normalizing the coming out process for LGB grandparents. Conversely, if adult children had negative attitudes toward homosexuality, they often forced their parents to maintain an illusion of heterosexuality for the grandchildren. "LGB grandparents who did not disclose or remained secretive did so to prevent becoming estranged from their families of origin… their sense of familialism was stronger than their need to disclose their individual identity" (Stelle, Fruhauf, Orel, & Landry-Meyer, 2010, p. 700).

Orel and Fruhauf's (2006) research with lesbian and bisexual grandmothers found that those grandmothers who did not disclose their sexual orientation to their grandchildren experienced this nondisclosure as being extremely stressful. Conversely, lesbian and bisexual grandmothers who were open and honest about their sexual orientation to their grandchildren increased the intergenerational connection and sense of social support that they had with their grandchildren. Gay grandfathers reported that it was easier coming out to their grandchildren than coming out to their own children and that the coming out process was more natural compared to the experience of coming out to their own children and immediate family members (Fruhauf, Orel, & Jenkins, 2009). This ease in coming out to their grandchildren was related to LGB grandparent's personal history of disclosing his or her sexual orientation with favorable results (Fruhauf, Orel, & Jenkins, 2009).

Collectively, the research on LGB grandparents indicates that managing disclosure about sexual orientation was the primary issue and that the decision to disclose or remain closeted was influenced by their perceptions of the level of sexism, heterosexism, and homonegativity within their particular setting and reflected their familial and societal relationships over time. All LGBT individuals struggle with decisions related to coming out, but LGB grandparents are unique in that their decisions are influenced by their adult children (Orel & Fruhauf, 2015). The research on LGB grandparents (Fruhauf et al., 2009; Orel, 2006) indicates that all LGB grandparents reported that their adult children played a major role in coming out to their grandchildren and LGB grandparents who did not reveal their sexual orientation did so to honor the request to remain secretive made by an adult child and/or to prevent becoming estranged from their families of origin. The need for LGB grandparents to maintain a strong connection to their families of origin is evident and many of the LGB grandparents indicated that this connection would be especially important if they required personal care in the future.

Within the general population, older adults with limitations in physical and/or cognitive functioning most often depend upon adult children, spouses, or other family members (e.g., grandchildren) for care, support and assistance. Traditionally, when care is needed by an LGBT older adult, it is usually the LGBT elder's significant other or partner who provides care (Fredriksen-Golden et al., 2011). Research indicates that LGBT older adults prefer to receive care from members of their families of choice instead of from members of their biological families (Hash, 2009; Heaphy, 2009; Price, 2011). If the LGBT older adult is single, or if his or her partner is unable or unwilling to provide care, then it would be expected that biological family members would be asked to provide it (Fredriksen-Goldsen et al., 2011). However, Fredriksen-Golden and colleagues (2011) found that only 11% of LGBT older adults actually received care directly from a biological family member. Limited research indicates that many LGBT older adults are hesitant to accept assistance from biological family members, especially if these familial relationships are distant or strained across their life course (Scherrer & Fedor, 2015). Other LGBT older adults may be hesitant to ask for caregiving assistance from biological family members if they fear that their sexual orientation or gender identity would be discovered and not accepted and honored.

The provision of caregiving assistance may also include making medical decisions for individuals. For LGBT older adults who have not established legal documents regarding who can make these medical or end-of-life decisions, the health care system will follow legal kinship definitions, which may exclude LGBT patients' health care wishes and/or the importance of including LGBT older adults' significant others in the decision-making process. Despite the importance of advance care planning, few LGBT older adults have completed such documentation (Scherrer & Fedor, 2015; MetLife, 2010). However, because LGBT older adults are twice as likely to live alone and more than four times as likely to be childless as heterosexual older adults (Espinoza, 2011), the majority of LGBT older adults have considered the importance of developing social support systems and alternative forms of family.

FAMILIES OF CHOICE

The literature on the LGBT population routinely identifies families of choice and chosen families to describe kin networks that LGBT individuals form. Families of choice and chosen families develop out of necessity when LGBT individuals become estranged from their biological families and/or if their biological families do not provide the needed support and care that one would expect from families. According to Price (2011), it is "in the absence of traditional, biological, support systems, gay men and lesbian women have embraced the need to develop and maintain diverse and, arguably, unique networks of support" (p. 1297).

Families of choice usually include partners and friends but may also include coworkers, neighbors, and ex-partners. To be considered a member of one's family of choice, members must provide many of the same supportive functions (e.g., emotional support, instrumental support) as would be expected from a member of one's family of origin (de Vries & Megathlin, 2009). However, "lesbians and gay men consider friendships as equally, or sometimes as even more important, than relationships with partners or relatives" (Heaphy, 2009, p. 129). However, research has shown that friendship networks vary among LGBT individuals throughout the life course. Lesbians are more likely to have close friendships with other lesbians and heterosexual women, whereas gay men are more likely to have gay or bisexual men in their friendship networks (Claassan, 2005; Grossman, D'Augelli, & Harshberger, 2000; Quam & Whitford, 1992). Bisexual individuals include more heterosexuals within their social networks and transgender older adults' friendship networks are more variable and often rely on support from Internet communities (Persson, 2009).

Chosen families are "flexible but often strong and supportive networks of friends, lovers, and even family of origin which provide the framework for the development of mutual care, responsibility, and commitment for many lesbians and gay men" (Weeks, Heaphy, & Donovan, 2001, p. 44). Chosen families are not "pretend" families or "surrogate" families, but instead are composed of individuals who provide emotional and practical support, with an emphasis on mutuality and reciprocity (Heaphy, 2009).

LGBT COMMUNITY

Another key source of social support for LGBT older adults is the LGBT community. Quam and Whitford (1992) concluded that successful aging for LGBT older adults requires a strong engagement with the LGBT community. Conversely, Jenkins, Walker, Cohen, and Curry (2010) reported that "older lesbian and gay individuals do not need to be involved in their lesbian and gay community to experience life satisfaction" (p. 415). While these researchers differ on the significance of the LGBT community for LGBT older adults, given the limited social networks for LGBT elders, many LGBT elders may want to become involved with the LGBT community.

Involvement within the LGBT community and the cohort to which they belong can vary based on the LGBT older adults' needs at a particular point in their life course. For example, LGBT older adults who represent the youngest cohort of baby boomer LGBT older adults will probably be actively involved in the LGBT community because it is this group of LGBT elders who were highly involved in the civil rights, feminist, and antiwar movements of the 60s and 70s

(Barker, Herdt, & de Vries, 2006). Additionally, it is this group that was actively involved in establishing volunteer programs and services addressing the needs of gay men who were living with HIV/AIDS. Conversely, LGBT older adults who are currently aged 75 and older may be facing physical and/or cognitive limitations that may restrict their active involvement in the LGBT community.

Research has also shown that the LGBT community in general has catered to a young cohort of LGBT individuals. Ageism exists within the LGBT community and many LGBT elders do not feel welcomed within the LGBT community that focuses on LGBT youth (Brotman, Ryan, & Cormier, 2002). Cahill, South, and Spade (2000) reported that the LGBT community is more ageist than the general public, and Kimmel, Rose, Orel, and Greene (2006) indicated that "ageist attitudes within the LGBT community often go uncontested" (p. 13). Because "ageism, beauty, and youthfulness are values that reign supreme within most gay and lesbian communities" (Brotman, Ryan, & Cormier, 2002, p. 198), LGBT elders may have difficulties feeling accepted and affirmed in most community LGBT organizations.

SPECIALIZED SERVICES FOR LGBT ELDERS AND THEIR FAMILIES

To address the unique needs and concerns of LGBT older adults, many LGBT community organizations have been initiated to specifically focus on LGBT elders. Senior Action in a Gay Environment (SAGE) was initiated in 1977 by a small group of gay men in New York City who were interested in addressing the needs of homebound older gay men and lesbians. Since its beginning, SAGE has been involved in building a sense of community for LGBT older adults. The mission of SAGE has evolved since 1977 and is now known as Services and Advocacy for GLBT Elders (SAGE). Currently, SAGE provides extensive and comprehensive training programs designed to sensitize social service providers to the unique needs and concerns of LGBT older adults as well as advocacy, programs, and services for LGBT older adults nationally. Most importantly, SAGE functions as an intergenerational organization; membership is open to everyone, regardless of age, encouraging intergenerational collaborations and social activities.

In 2010, SAGE was awarded funding by the U.S. Administration on Aging (AOA) to establish the National Resource Center for LGBT Aging, marking the first time that the AOA acknowledged that the unique needs and concerns of older LGBT individuals must be addressed. The National Resource Center for LGBT Aging provides information, assistance, and resources for both aging network providers and LGBT organizations. Websites of the National Resource

Center for LGBT Aging (www.lgbtagingcenter.org), the National Center for Lesbian Rights (www.nclrights.org), local LGBT community centers, and HIV/AIDS service organizations, provide information on best practices that specifically target LGBT older adults and/or LGBT caregivers and they provide timely information on the unique needs and concerns of LGBT older adults. These websites are useful places to start, with additional information on innovative evidence-based programs for LGBT older adults and their families available through the LGBT Aging Project (Fenway Health, n.d.), the AOA (n.d.), and the National LGBT Health Education Center (www.lgbthealtheducation.org). These nonprofit organizations have collaborated with aging network providers and LGBT community organizations to provide professional training that would increase public awareness on the issues that impact the lives of LGBT older adults and their families and developed strategies that would improve services.

TRENDS AND FUTURE RESEARCH

The personal experiences of LGBT older adults have been characterized by isolation, social stigma, and systematic discrimination. These factors have shaped LGBT older adults' thinking and behaviors and may continue to affect their well-being into later years. LGBT older adults have experienced numerous challenges within a heterosexist society, but they have also developed unique strengths and resilience that have allowed them to lead rewarding lives in difficult circumstances. Most importantly, LGBT older adults have established unique families and social support networks that have assisted them in meeting the challenges of aging.

With the general increase in the older adult population, it is also assumed that the number of LGBT individuals reaching later adulthood will significantly increase in number and proportion (Orel, 2014). Although accurate estimates of the LGBT older adult population are not available, it is estimated that by 2030, four million Americans aged 65 and older will be LGBT (Hunter, 2005). With the dramatic increase in the LGBT older adult population, it is imperative that the importance of "family" relationships and social support systems be addressed, particularly through research exploring the effect of parents' sexual orientation on children (Neville & Henrickson, 2008).

It is evident that there is no typical family form for any cultural group; thus there is no typical LGBT family. Future research must explore the unique experiences of LGBT older adults of color. Research on family roles, support, and structure indicates that there are variations based on racial background, ethnic identities, religious affiliations, social economic status, and national origin.

Additional research is needed to explore these variations among LGBT older adults' familial relationships and social support systems, particularly among families of older bisexual and transgender individuals. According to Cohler (2005), "there has been very little study of men and women who self-define as bisexual in a continuing preference across the course of life" (p. 87). Too often, the lives of bisexual elders are only examined in comparison with lesbian and gay older adults (Dworkin, 2006; Rodriguez-Rust, 2012).

LGBT older adults reflect the diversity of the general population. However, research that has been conducted on LGBT older adults tends to focus on the LGBT populations that are part of the dominant discourse (e.g., able bodied, able minded, White, middle class, European American, and female or male). Research on LGBT older adults requires greater attention to the diversity that exists within the LGBT older adult population and the intersectionality of age, gender, religion, national origin, sexual orientation, socioeconomic status, ethnicity and race, and degree of physical ability and cognitive ability over the life course (Orel & Fruhauf, 2015).

It is important to recognize that the oldest LGBT elders (e.g., aged 75 and older) were raised in the early days of radio, television, telephone, and audio recordings. Older LGBT adults aged 60 to 75 most likely were raised with televisions in their living rooms, and they witnessed the introduction of personal computers and the advent of the Internet. Conversely, LGBT individuals under the age of 60 are experiencing many new forms of communication (e.g., Facebook, Twitter), the power of mass communication for advocacy, and the ability to legally marry prior to reaching later adulthood. LGBT older adults over the age of 75 grew up believing that homosexuality was a sickness, amoral, and criminal. In contrast, current LGBT adults have witnessed the Supreme Court decision that affords the rights of marriage to same-sex couples and homosexuality is no longer considered a psychopathological disorder. There are numerous empirical articles and books that highlight the interpersonal strength and resiliency of the LGBT older adult population (see Fredriksen-Goldsen et al., 2013; Orel & Fruhauf, 2015). Research specifically exploring the unique strengths of LGBT older adults and their ability to develop strong social support systems, positive coping strategies, and resilience is needed.

Research is also needed to explore the impact of disclosing one's sexual orientation and gender identity across generational cohorts of LGBT older adults. With the repeal of "don't ask, don't tell" and the legalization of same-sex marriages, the culture has now created a disclosure imperative, whereby LGBT individuals are expected to be open and honest about their sexual orientation with friends, family, neighbors, and colleagues. For some LGBT older adults, this disclosure imperative may be problematic when one takes into consideration their generational memories. It has only been 46 years since the Stonewall Rebellion of 1969 when gay men "openly declared their sexual identity as something good while criticizing American society for its intolerance" (Seidman, 2002, p. 64). Until American society declares that homosexuality and aging and the aged are to be valued, LGBT older adults may continue to struggle with the issue of disclosure, especially when they assume roles (e.g., grandparent) that have been identified as key "family" milestones that historically only heterosexual older adults experience.

Previous research has indicated that many preliberation LGBT elders (e.g., those born and raised prior to the gay liberation) internalized the discriminatory attitudes of an intolerant society (Kaufman & Raphael, 1996). Brotman, Ryan, and Cormier (2002) found that LGBT elders who did not challenge these internalized negative heterosexist beliefs experienced higher rates of depression, stress, addictions, and suicide. LGBT older adults who internalized the discriminatory attitudes of both a heterosexist and ageist society would find themselves struggling with their self-identity as being both LGBT and old. Ideally, the majority of LGBT elders would have deconstructed the negative images associated with heterosexism and ageism and developed adaptive coping skills and strategies. These LGBT elders would demonstrate psychological resilience and would be able to age successfully with strong levels of life satisfaction, low self-criticism, and few psychosomatic complaints. As this chapter has illustrated, the quality and extent of affirming family and social support networks is related to LGBT elders' own level of comfort with their sexual orientation (Herdt, Beeler, & Rawls, 1997). Therefore, it will require an affirming culture that recognizes the strengths and resiliency of the LGBT older adult population so that they can age with dignity and our collective support and respect.

REFERENCES

Adams, K., Sanders, S., & Auth, E. (2004). Loneliness and depression in independent living retirement communities: Risk and resilience factors. *Aging and Mental Health, 8*, 475–485.

Ajrouch, K., Blandon, A., & Antonucci, T. (2005). Social networks among men and women: The effects of age and socioeconomic status. *Journals of Gerontology Series B-Psychological Sciences and Social Services, 60*, S311–S317.

Barker, J., Herdt, G., & de Vries, B. (2006). Social support in the lives of lesbians and gay men in midlife and later. *Sexuality Research and Social Policy, 3*, 1–23.

Berkman, L. F., & Glass, T. (2000). Social integration, social networks, social support, and health. In L. F. Berkman & I. Kawachi (Eds.), *Social epidemiology* (pp. 137–173). New York, NY: Oxford University Press.

Brotman, S., Ryan, B., & Cormier, R. (2002). The health and social service needs of gay and lesbian elders and their families in Canada. *The Gerontologist, 43*(2), 192–202.

Cahill, S., South, K., & Spade, J. (2000). *Outing age: Public policy issues affecting gay, lesbian, bisexual, and transgender elders.* New York, NY: The Policy Institute of the National Gay and Lesbian Task Force Foundation.

Cicirelli, V. (2010). Attachment relationships in old age. *Journal of Social and Personal Relationships, 27*, 191–199.

Claassan, C. (2005). *Whistling women: A study of the lives of older lesbians.* New York, NY: The Haworth Press.

Cohler, B. J. (2005). Life course social science perspectives on the GLBT family. *Journal of GLBT Family Studies, 1*, 69–95.

Connidis, I. (2010). *Family ties and aging*. Thousand Oaks, CA: Sage.

Conway, F., Magai, C., Jones, S., Fiori, K., & Gillespie, M. (2013). A six-year follow-up study of social network changes among African-American, Caribbean, and U.S. born Caucasian urban older adults. *International Journal of Aging and Human Development, 76*, 1–27.

Cook-Daniels, L. (2015). Transgender aging: What practitioners should know. In N. Orel & C. Fruhauf (Eds.), *The lives of LGBT older adults: Understanding challenges and resilience* (pp. 193–215). Washington, DC: American Psychological Association.

Cornwell, B., Laumann, E., & Schumm, L. (2008). The social connectedness of older adults: A national profile. *American Sociological Review, 73*, 185–203.

Cotton, S., Anderson, W., & McCullough, B. (2013). Impact of internet use on loneliness and contact with others among older adults: Cross sectional analysis. *Journal of Medical Internet Research, 15*, 39.

Cronin, A., Ward, R., Pugh, S., King, A., & Price, E. (2011). Categories and their consequences: Understanding and supporting the caring relationships of older lesbians, gay and bisexual people. *International Social Work, 54*, 421–435.

Demo, D., Allen, K., & Fine, M. (2000). *Handbook of family diversity*. New York, NY: Oxford University Press.

de Vries, B., & Megathlin, D. (2009). The meaning of friendship for gay men and lesbians in the second half of life. *Journal of GLBT Family Studies, 5*, 82–98.

Doubova, S., Perez-Cuevas, R., Espinosa-Alcron, P., & Flores-Hernadez, S. (2010). Social network types and functional dependency in older adults in Mexico. *BMC Public Health, 10*(104), 1–10.

Dworkin, S. (2006). The aging bisexual: The invisible of the invisible minority. In D. Kimmel, T. Rose, & S. David (Eds.), *Lesbian, gay, bisexual and transgender aging: Research and clinical perspectives* (pp. 36–52). New York, NY: Columbia University Press.

Erosheva, E., Kim, H., Emlet, C., & Fredriksen-Goldsen, K. (2015). Social networks of lesbian, gay, bisexual, and transgender older adults. *Research on Aging, 38*(1), 98–123.

Espinoza, R. (2011). The diverse elder coalition and LGBT aging: Connecting communities, issues, and resources in a historic moment. *Public Policy and Aging Report, 21*, 8–12.

Fenway Health. (n.d.). *LGBT Aging Project*. Retrieved from http://fenwayhealth.org/the-fenway-institute/lgbt-aging-project

Fiori, K., Smith, J., & Antonucci, T. (2007). Social network types among older adults: A multidimensional approach. *The Journals of Gerontology Series B: Psychological Sciences and Social Sciences, 62*, P322–P330.

Fredricksen-Goldsen, K. (2009). Older GLBT family and community life: Contemporary experiences, realities, and future directions (forward for special edition). *Journal of GLBT Family Studies, 5*(1–2), 2–4.

Fredriksen-Goldsen, K., Emlet, C., Kim, H., Muraco, A., Erosheva, E., Goldsen, J., et al. (2013). The physical and mental health of lesbian, gay male, and bisexual older adults: The role of key health indicators and risk and protective factors. *The Gerontologist, 53*, 664–675.

Fredriksen-Goldsen. K., Kim, H., Emlet, C., Muraco, A., Erosheva, E., Hoy-Ellis, C., et al. (2011). *The aging and health report: Disparities and resilience among lesbian, gay, bisexual, and transgender older adults*. Seattle, WA: Institute for Multigenerational Health.

Fruhauf, C., Orel, N., & Jenkins, D. (2009). The coming out process of gay grandfathers: Perceptions of their adult children's influence. *Journal of GLBT Family Studies, 5*, 99–118.

Fullmer, E. (2006). Lesbian, gay, bisexual, and transgender aging. In D. Morrow & L. Messinger (Eds.), *Sexual orientation & gender expression in social work practice: Working with gay, lesbian, bisexual, and transgender people* (pp. 284–303). New York, NY: Columbia University Press.

Glass, T., & Balfour, J. (2003). Neighborhoods, aging, and functional limitations. In I. Kawachi & L. Berkman (Eds.), *Neighborhoods and health* (pp. 303–334). Oxford, England: Oxford University Press.

Goldberg, A. (2010). *Lesbian and gay parents and their children: Research on the family life cycle*. Washington, DC: American Psychological Association.

Gray, A. (2009). The social capital of older people. *Ageing and Society, 29*, 5–31.

Grossman, A., D'Augelli, A., & Harshberger, S. (2000). Social support networks of lesbian, gay, bisexual adults 60 years of age and older. *The Journal of Gerontology: Series B, Psychological Sciences and Social Sciences, 55B*, 171–179.

Grossman, A., D'Augelli, A., & O'Connell, T. (2001). Being lesbian, gay, bisexual, and 60 or older in North America. *Journal of Gay and Lesbian Social Services, 13*, 23–40.

Hasenbush, A., Flores, A., Kastanis, A., Sears, B., & Gates, G. (2014). *The LGBT divide: A data portrait of LGBT people in the midwestern, mountain, and southern states*. The Williams Institute. Retrieved from http://williamsinstitute.law.ucla.edu/research/lgbt-divide-dec-2014

Hash, K. (2009). Caregiving and post-caregiving experiences of midlife and older gay men and lesbians. *Journal of Gerontological Social Work, 47*, 121–138.

Heaphy, B. (2009). Choice and its limits in older lesbian and gay narratives of relational life. *Journal of GLBT Family Studies, 5*, 119–138.

Herdt, G., Beeler, J., & Rawls, T. (1997). Life course diversity among older lesbians and gay men: A study in Chicago. *Journal of Gay, Lesbian, and Bisexual Identity, 2*, 199–230.

Hunter, S. (2005). *Midlife and older LGBT adults: Knowledge and affirmative practice for the social sciences*. Binghamton, NY: Haworth Press.

Hurlbert, J., & Acock, A. (1990). The effects of marital-status on the form and composition of social networks. *Social Science Quarterly, 71*, 163–174.

Jenkins, D., Walker, C., Cohen, H., & Curry, L. (2010). A lesbian older adult managing identity disclosure: A case study. *Journal of Gerontological Social Work, 53*(5), 402–420.

Kaufman, G., & Raphael, L. (1996). *Coming out of shame: Transforming gay and lesbian lives*. New York, NY: Doubleday.

Kimmel, D., Rose, T., Orel, N., & Greene, B. (2006). Historical context for research on lesbian, gay, bisexual, and transgender aging. In D. Kimmel, T. Rose, & S. David (Eds.), *Lesbian, gay, bisexual, and transgender aging* (pp. 1–19). New York, NY: Columbia University Press.

LGBT Community Center of Greater Cleveland. (2015). *LGBT older adults health and wellness report: A survey of LGBT older adults in Northwest Ohio*. Cleveland, OH: Author.

Litwin, H., & Landau, R. (2000). Social network type and social support among the old-old. *Journal of Aging Studies, 14*(2), 213–228.

Litwin, H., & Shiovitz-Ezra, S. (2011). Social network type and subjective well being in a national sample of older Americans. *The Gerontologist, 51*, 379–388.

McLaughlin, D., Vagenas, D., Pachana, N., Begum, N., & Dobson, A. (2010). Gender differences in social network size and satisfaction in adults in their 70s. *The Journal of Health Psychology, 15*, 671–679.

Metlife. (2010). *Still out, still aging: The MetLife study of lesbian, gay, bisexual, and transgender baby boomers*. New York, NY: Author.

Morrow, D. (2006). Coming out as gay, lesbian, bisexual, and transgender. In D. F. Morrow & L. Messinger (Eds.), *Sexual orientation and gender expression in social work practice: Working with gays, lesbian, bisexual, and transgender people* (pp. 129–149). New York, NY: Columbia University Press.

Nardi, P. (1999). *Gay men's friendships: Invincible communities*. Chicago, IL: Chicago University Press.

Neville, S., & Henrickson, M. (2008). The constitution of 'lavender families': A LGB perspective. *Journal of Clinical Nursing, 18*, 849–856.

Orel, N. (2004). Gay, lesbian, bisexual elders: Expressed needs and concerns across focus groups. *Journal of Gerontological Social Work, 43*(2–3), 57–77.

Orel, N. (2006). Lesbian and bisexual women as grandparents: The centrality of sexual orientation in the grandparent-grandchild relationship. In D. Kimmel, T. Rose, & S. David (Eds.), *Lesbian, gay, bisexual, and transgender aging: Research and clinical perspectives* (pp. 173–194). New York, NY: Columbia University Press.

Orel, N. (2014). Investigating the needs and concerns of lesbian, gay, bisexual, and transgender older adults: The use of qualitative and quantitative methodology. *Journal of Homosexuality, 61*, 53–78.

Orel, N., & Fruhauf, C. (2006). Lesbian and bisexual grandmothers' perceptions of the grandparent-grandchild relationship. *Journal of GLBT Family Studies, 2*(1), 43–70.

Orel, N., & Fruhauf, C. (2013). Lesbian, gay, bisexual, and transgender grandparenting. In A. Goldberg & K. Allen (Eds.), *LGBT parent families: Possibilities for new research and implications for practice* (pp. 177–192). New York, NY: Springer Publishing.

Orel, N., & Fruhauf, C. (2015). *The lives of LGBT older adults and their families: Understanding challenges and resilience.* Washington, DC: American Psychological Association.

Ozbay, F., Johnson, D., Dimoulas, E., Morgan, C., Charney, D., & Southwick, S. (2007). Social support and resilience to stress: From neurobiology to clinical practices. *Psychiatry, 4*(5), 35–40.

Persson, D. (2009). Unique challenges of transgender aging: Implications from the literature. *Journal of Gerontological Social Work, 52*, 633–646.

Price, E. (2011). Caring for mum and dad: Lesbian women negotiating family and navigating care. *British Journal of Social Work, 41*, 1288–1303.

Quam, J., & Whitford, G. (1992). Adaptation and age-related expectations of older gay and lesbian adults. *The Gerontologist, 32*, 367–374.

Rodriguez-Rust, P. (2012). Aging in the bisexual community. In T. Witten & E. Eyler (Eds.), *Gay, lesbian, bisexual and transgender aging: Challenges in research, practice, and policy* (pp. 162–186). Baltimore, MD: Johns Hopkins University Press.

Scherrer, K., & Fedor, J. (2015). Family issues for LGBT older adults. In N. Orel & C. Fruhauf (Eds.), *The lives of LGBT older adults: Understanding challenges and resilience* (pp. 171–192). Washington, DC: American Psychological Association.

Seidman, S. (2002). *Beyond the closet: The transformation of gay and lesbian life*. New York, NY: Routledge.

Smith, P., & Drew, L. (2002). Grandparenthood. In M. Bernstein (Ed.), *Handbook of parenting, Vol. 3: Being and becoming a parent* (2nd ed., pp. 141–172). Mahwah, NJ: Lawrence Erlbaum Associates.

Stelle, C., Fruhauf, C., Orel, N., & Landry-Meyer, L. (2010). Grandparenting in the 21st century: Issues of diversity in grandparent-grandchild relationships. *Journal of Gerontological Social Work, 53*, 682–701.

Tasker, F. (2013). Lesbian and gay parenting post-heterosexual divorce and separation. In A. Goldberg & K. Allen (Eds.), *LGBT parent families: Implications in research and implications for practice* (pp. 3–20). New York, NY: Springer Publishing.

Townsend. P. (1957). *The family life of old people*. New York, NY: Routledge.

U.S. Administration on Aging. (n.d.). *A toolkit for serving diverse communities*. Retrieved from www.aoa.acl.gov/AoA_Programs/Tools_Resources/DOCS/AoA_DiversityToolkit_full.pdf

Weeks, J., Heaphy, B., & Donovan, C. (2001). *Same sex intimacies: Families of choice and other life experiments*. New York, NY: Routledge.

Weston, K. (1997). *Families we choose: Lesbians, gays, kinship*. New York, NY: Columbia University Press.

Witten, T. (2009). Graceful exits: Intersection of aging, transgender identities, and the family/community. *Journal of GLBT Family Studies, 5*(1–2), 35–61.

Witten, T., & Eyler, A. (2012). Transgender and aging: Beings and becomings. In T. Witten & Eyler (Eds.), *Gay, lesbian, bisexual, and transgender aging: Challenges in research, practice, and policy* (pp. 187–269). Baltimore, MD: Johns Hopkins Press.

Woolwine, D. (2000). Community in gay male experience and moral discourse. *Journal of Homosexuality, 38*(4), 5–37.

Wrzus, C., Hanel, M., Wagner, J., & Neyer, F. (2013). Social network changes and life events across the life span: A meta-analysis. *Psychological Bulletin, 139*, 53–80.

CHAPTER 8

Aging LGBT Military Service Members and Veterans

Mariann Mankowski

ABSTRACT

The purpose of this chapter is to highlight the experiences and needs of aging sexual and gender minority (SGM) veterans. Significant demographic changes in the composition of aging military veterans have taken place. Most noticeably since the repeal of "don't ask, don't tell" attention has been drawn to this population of older veterans and their specific mental, physical, and psychosocial health care needs. Recent policy, program, and research initiatives have begun to address the significant health disparities of this population of older adults. SGM veterans are more likely to report higher rates of sexual harassment and sexual assault, and are more vulnerable to homelessness and unemployment when compared to the general population of older lesbian, gay, bisexual, and transgender (LGBT) adults. Aging SGM veterans may also carry a heavy burden as a result of their experiences as service members and may be reticent to disclose their sexual identity with formal veteran service programs. Access to and utilization of social care networks and social support for SGM aging veterans is a serious concern. Isolation, poorer health outcomes, and increased chronic health conditions may exacerbate the marginalization this older adult population has experienced. A majority of SGM veterans will utilize community-based services, and it is essential that all health care professionals understand the unique needs

http://dx.doi.org/10.1891/0198-8794.37.111

of this cohort of older adults. Future directions for research, policy, education, and service delivery are explored.

INTRODUCTION

Military veterans over the age of 65 comprise an estimated 43% of the current U.S. veteran population (U.S. Census Bureau, 2012; U.S. Department of Veterans Affairs, 2015). The Office of Disease Control and Health Prevention (2014) report, *Healthy People 2020* acknowledged the need for research on the health of sexual and gender minorities (SGMs), and recent reports from the Institute of Medicine (IOM, 2011), the Veterans Health Administration (VHA), and the Joint Commission on Veterans Affairs (2011) have identified research gaps and opportunities for improving lesbian, gay, bisexual, and transgender (LGBT) health. This chapter highlights the needs of SGM aging veterans, describes the importance of social care networks and social support, identifies health disparities and signature health issues for this aging population, and discusses potential program and research needs as well as future psychosocial, mental, and physical health directions of older SGM veterans.

BACKGROUND

LGBT persons have served in the military throughout history despite military policies that necessitated concealment of their sexual orientation. Recent demographic reports estimate there are approximately 71,000 active duty, ready reserve, and standby reserve SGM service members in today's military and approximately one million SGM military veterans (Gates, 2010). In addition, recent Department of Defense (DOD) estimates show that there are approximately 15,000 transgender military personal currently serving in all branches of the military and 134,000 transgender veterans (Gates & Herman, 2014).

The VHA is the largest health provider in the world and may be one of the largest health care providers for SGM individuals. Until recently, VHA policies have historically aligned with U.S. DOD policies, whereby sexual orientation was neither acknowledged nor identified by providers or in medical records, limiting health care data, and possibly the quality of care to SGM veterans. In 2012, the VHA created the Office of Health Equity focusing on the health care needs of LGBT veterans and made SGM veteran health care a systemwide priority (Lehavot & Simpson, 2012). Comprehensive changes in systemwide medical records may be forthcoming and current omnibus bills in the Senate would extend VHA services for Iraq and Afghanistan veterans from 5 years to 15 years postdeployment. This policy change may have positive ramifications for aging SGM veterans.

America's long-standing prohibition of lesbian, gay, and bisexual service members was modified in 1994 under the National Defense Authorization Act, more commonly known as "don't ask, don't tell" (DADT; Moran, 2013). From 1994–2010, DADT formally changed discharge authorization based on *sexual orientation* to discharge based on *sexual behavior* (Cochran, Balsam, Flentje, Malte, & Simpson, 2013). Between 1980 and 2009, approximately 27,000 LGBT service members experienced sexual minority based discharge (approximately 13,000 during DADT; Gates, 2010). In 2010, DADT was repealed, yet discharge based on sexual behavior is still possible under Article 134 of the Uniform Code of Military Justice (UCMJ). UCMJ gives the military broad power to order discharges for any service member behaving in a manner seen prejudicial to "good order and discipline" (10 U.S.C.934 art 134; 2010). Fear of expulsion, discrimination, and stigma may predominate SGM veterans' experiences with the military (including the VHA), whereby their reticence to utilize physical, mental, and support services may be explained. The underreported victimization many SGM service members experienced from their "brothers in arms" may also deter many aging SGM veterans from accessing care from formal military-related institutions, which may have long-term negative consequences for SGM veterans.

MINORITY STRESS MODEL

Research on stress indicates members from disadvantaged social groups, including women, are especially vulnerable, reporting higher depression and related stress scores than women who are married, older, and maintain higher socioeconomic status (Thoits, 1995a, 1995b). Accordingly, Frayne et al. (2006) note that exposure to combat and military sexual trauma (MST) and harassment are associated with poor health in women veterans and may contribute to potentially higher medical and mental health utilization rates in the near future. Meyer (2003), in the Minority Stress Model, hypothesized that being a member of a disenfranchised group that faced discrimination, stigma, and the threat of potential violence creates opportunities for stress and internalized stigma. According to Herek (2007), social stigma may result in SGM's experience of denigration, disempowerment, and feelings of marginalization.

Previous military research has noted the importance of unit cohesion as a buffering mechanism for the negative effects of war (Figley, 1978; Kulka et al., 1990). Figley (1978) suggested the more stressful the event such as that experienced at war, the greater the need for support. Fontana, Rosenheck, and Horvath (1997) using the National Vietnam Veterans Readjustment Survey (NVVRS) concluded that low social support may perpetuate mental distress symptoms in those exposed to severe trauma. Recent studies have begun to identify the negative effects DADT (and previous military policies) have had on SGM veterans (Blosnich, Bossarte, & Silenzio, 2012; Burks, 2011; Mattocks, et al., 2013a, 2013b; Moradi, 2009). These studies suggest forced concealment has created undo stressors related to fear of discharge, loss of employment, as well as victimizations.

SOCIAL CARE NETWORKS AND SOCIAL SUPPORT

Social care networks, social support, and quality of life indicators of SGM veterans are of critical importance, and knowledge of the experience of aging SGM veterans is essential if we are to provide services to this cohort of aging veterans. Most veterans, regardless of age, do not utilize VHA services, and given the previous ban of SGM from the military and service academies, SGM veterans may also be reluctant to utilize VHA services (Haskell et al., 2011; Mattocks et al., 2013a; Simpson, Balsam, Cochran, Lehavot, & Gold, 2013; Yano et al., 2011). Therefore, it is incumbent on community-based health care providers to become aware of the needs of this population.

Social care networks and social support have been extensively studied relative to health outcomes, yet little is known about SGM veterans' access to and utilization of social care networks and social support. Physical and mental health outcomes have been associated with social care networks and social support (Brennan-Ing et al., 2014). Over the past several decades studies have noted the importance of social support in the quality of life of aging individuals (Cotten & Skinner, 2000; Frayne et al., 2006; Fredriksen-Goldsen et al., 2014; Tucker & Kelley, 2009). Fredriksen-Goldsen et al. (2014) found social support and social care network size to be positively associated with quality of life outcomes and Fredriksen-Goldsen et al. (2012) identified SGM individuals in the general population reported less social support and smaller social care networks. Therefore, protective factors such as social support and social networks may also be limited for aging SGM veterans.

Of particular importance are the social care networks and social support utilized by SGM veterans as they age. Social care networks are identified as dynamic and multifaceted resources used by individuals to assist in activities of daily living (ADLs), enhance quality of life, and maintain relational connections over the life span (Cohen & Syme, 1985; House & Kahn, 1985; Wills, 1985). Social support includes the relational (someone to talk with, share a meal, etc.), functional (drive to appointment, help with house care, etc.), and instrumental (housing vouchers, food stamps, health insurance) support individuals receive throughout their daily lives (Cohen, Hettler, & Park, 1997; Cohen & Syme, 1985; House & Kahn, 1985; Thoits, 1995a, 1995b; Wills, 1985).

The ramifications of the lack of social support and its negative correlation to physical and mental health outcomes including increased mortality rates have also been examined (Mankowski, Mattocks, Haskell, & Brandt, 2015; Mattocks et al., 2012; Thoits, 1995b). According to Basham (2008), social support can be a "central protective factor" (or buffer) in alleviating the effects of military trauma. In the general population, social isolation has been linked to poor mental and physical health outcomes, higher levels of cognitive impairment, and premature death and disease (Ailshire & Crimmins, 2011). The recent study by Brennan-Ing, Seidel, Larson, and Karpiak (2014) identified significant gaps in the literature on the service needs of LGBT individuals and offered important population-based information on social care networks and social support of the aging veteran SGM population. Previous studies by Brennan-Ing et al. (2014) found many LGBT older adults do not rely on LGBT-focused organizations to meet their needs, and most rely on mainstream providers.

The buffering hypothesis suggests that social supports may ameliorate the effects of stressful, chronic discrimination, harassment, and potential violence. Social supports and social care networks may help in redefining the harmful potential of a situation, reduce or eliminate negative affective reactions to a stressful event, and/or alleviate the impact of stress. Aging has been associated with a reduction in social care networks and social supports, and sexual minorities have been identified as maintaining smaller, nonfamilial social supports and social care networks across the life span (Brennan-Ing et al., 2014; Fredriksen-Goldsen et al., 2014). Therefore, SGM veterans may be vulnerable to having smaller social care networks and reduced social support as they age due to their previous experience with military policies that required concealment and denial of their sexual orientation. Finally, as noted previously, chronic stress and anxiety as experienced by SGM veterans may be additional factors associated with compromised immune systems.

Women and men differ in the types of structural support they have (Thoits, 1995b). Men frequently have larger social networks that are less intensive, whereas women's networks are less extensive but more intensive (Thoits, 1995b). Studies also show differences in the level of perceived social support by age, marital status, and socioeconomic status (Thoits, 1995a, 1995b). Additionally, Everett, Hall, and Hamilton-Mason (2010) raise the important issue of "contagion of stress" suggesting that social support may not buffer racial minorities against stress if members of their social network also experience chronic and acute stress conditions. Brennan-Ing et al. (2014) found gay men reported limited social care networks and greater vulnerability for isolation.

SGM HEALTH CARE NEEDS

Health Disparities

Significant health disparities and at-risk behaviors of some LGBT veterans have been identified, including diabetes, chronic heart disease, smoking, substance use, and obesity (Fredriksen-Goldsen et al., 2012). The intersection of veteran status, aging, and SGM orientation may place LGBT veterans at an even higher risk for long term mental and physical health disparities. To date, LGBT health research remains an under studied topic, and the gap in our knowledge of health indicators for aging SGM veterans is particularly large.

The nexus of health disparities among SGM veterans is complex, multidimensional, and intersects with age, race, gender, and urban/rural residence. These health disparities are evidenced across subpopulations of older adults and suggest veterans may be at higher risk than the general civilian population and their heterosexual military peers. As an at-risk subpopulation, aging SGM veterans are more likely to experience poor health, physical disabilities, lowered access to health care, less financial security, and more mental health stressors than their peers (Fredriksen-Goldsen et al., 2012). In addition to the aforementioned risk factors, SGM veterans are also at higher risk for suicide or suicidal ideation than the general population, and they are also more likely to have experienced trauma than civilian SGM individuals (Blosnich, Bossarte, & Silenzio, 2012). Whereby the risks to aging SGM veterans are significant. Recent reports from the VHA reveal that 70% of veterans who completed suicide were over the age of 50, two times the rate of the same civilian cohort.

Lesbian veterans have reported poorer health status and they are more likely to have experienced adverse childhood experiences than their civilian or heterosexual military peers (Lehavot & Simpson, 2012). Of particular note, as sexual minorities, lesbian and bisexual women are overrepresented in the military compared to the general population comprising approximately 43% of the military's sexual minorities (Lehavot & Simpson, 2012; Moradi, 2009). SGM female veterans are more likely to use tobacco and be obese and less physically mobile than either civilian women or heterosexual female veterans. SGM female veterans also are more likely to be diagnosed with anxiety, depression, posttraumatic stress, and substance use disorders (Blosnich, Foynes, & Shipherd, 2013; Blosnich & Silenzio, 2013). SGM female veterans also report a lifetime experience of sexual violence compared to heterosexual peers (Booth et al., 2012) and report a greater aversion to utilizing the VHA.

Gay male veterans are more likely to report low income, interpersonal isolation, and housing vulnerability than either their heterosexual male military peers or civilian males, which also has negative long-term consequences as veterans age

(Blosnich, Foynes, & Shipherd, 2013; Blosnich & Silenzio, 2013). Finally, Der-Martirosian, Cordasco, and Washington (2013) report that the rural population of veterans experiences greater prevalence of most diseases and lower health-related quality of life than urban veterans, putting them at higher risk for lowered quality of life and illness.

Military Stressors

In addition to military stress related to deployment, exposure to combat, and other hostile environments, military sexual trauma (MST) is a serious problem that has lifelong ramifications. SGM service members who experience stress and in particular MST are at greater risk for developing mental health problems than their heterosexual counterparts. According to recent preliminary Department of Veterans Affairs (VA) research, "MST leads to a 59% risk for mental health issues" (Mulhall, 2009, p. 9). Evidence indicates women who have experienced MST are more likely to suffer from depression, posttraumatic stress disorder (PTSD), and eating disorders than their peers who have not experienced MST (Defense Department Advisory Committee on Women in the Services, 2013; Mattocks et al., 2012). Utilizing the Veterans SF-36 health survey instrument (Ware, 1993), Frayne et al. (2006) found that women veterans had consistently worse scores than female nonveterans on the SF-36 "in every domain of physical and mental health" (p. S43).

Prevalence rates of MST vary from 5% to 71% among both male and female service members. The residual effects of sexual victimization are often expressed in somatic complaints as well and psychological distress leading to a cascade of mental and physical health care needs (Booth et al., 2012). Anxiety, depression, PTSD, and substance abuse as well as obesity, hypertension, chronic pain, and gastrointestinal complaints are several of the ramifications of sexual victimization (Mattocks et al., 2013b). Lifetime prevalence of sexual assault among SGM veterans suggests a greater risk for revictimization. Though unconfirmed and understudied, MST reports among SGM veterans and service members suggest SGM service members may be a targeted subpopulation because of their sexual orientation, resulting in higher rates of sexual victimization while in the military, resulting in lifelong psychosocial issues.

Harassment, prejudice, and concealment of sexual orientation are considered stressors that are deleterious to health and quality of life (Moradi, 2009). Concealment also creates the potential for isolation, preventing service members from relational connection, support, and protection against possible victimization and may in fact heighten vulnerability to internalized stigma and the negative consequences of victimization and discrimination. With regard to SGM aging veterans, the Minority Stress Model implies the importance of peer group affiliation as a protective feature against the onslaught of daily heterosexism and homophobia. Aging SGM veterans may have lacked this opportunity to develop peer group affiliation while in the military, and therefore may have been prevented from developing these connections as veterans.

Signature Mental Health Issues

Every military conflict has its own unique "signature injuries." For example, traumatic brain injuries are the signature injuries of the conflicts in Operation Iraqi Freedom (OIF) and Operation Enduring Freedom (OEF) in Iraq and Afghanistan respectively, while many service members from Operation Desert Storm presented with a cluster of respiratory illnesses subsequently identified as Gulf War syndrome. Agent Orange, an herbicide used by the U.S. military as a defoliant in Vietnam, caused a cluster of various diseases including cancers, skin diseases, and infertility issues, which became signature injuries of the Vietnam Era. Additionally, Vietnam veterans are twice as likely to suffer from PTSD than any other military cohort to date. They also experienced difficulty transitioning to civilian life due in part to the widespread opposition to the war, which may have resulted in further social isolation. According to the IOM (2008) "signature injuries" of military veterans include muscular skeletal disorders, pain disorders, chronic pulmonary and other heart conditions, and certain mental health disorders. Overall, aging veterans are also at higher risk for depression, suicide, mental and health issues, and reintegration difficulties as well as financial problems, intimate partner violence and family and marital discord (Mattocks et al., 2013b; Simpson et al., 2013).

Depressive symptoms are common in aging populations and cause both suffering and impairment that frequently go undiagnosed or untreated (Sanders, Comijs, Bremmer, Deeg, & Beekman, 2015; Unutzer, 2007). In general, depression in aging veterans co-occurs with physical illness creating increased risk for suicide. Depression may also lead to additional complications such as poor nutrition, sedentary lifestyle, and isolation (Sanders et al., 2015). Both aging and depression may also alter pain perception, whereby reduced levels of pain tolerance and increased utilization of pain medications may occur. Finally, the potential for increased health care costs may overburden an already challenged veteran population (Mattocks et al., 2013b).

A significant gap in the literature on the health related and psychosocial issues experienced by older female veterans suggests a need for continued research and program evaluation. Given health care providers awareness of the risk for social isolation, chronic health issues including pain, obesity, heart-related conditions, and the economic insecurity that frequently accompanies aging and retirement, they are uniquely positioned to provide care, services, and initiate research in these areas. Aging female SGM veterans often maintain the role of caregiver, whereby they may be at risk for ignoring or denying their own physical and mental health needs (Mattocks et al., 2013a).

The Clinical Evaluation Program (Stuart, Murray, Ursano, & Wright, 2002) reports women were more frequently diagnosed with mental disorders, musculoskeletal/connective tissue disorders, and ill-defined conditions. PTSD, depression, and hypertension were the three most prevalent health issues facing female veterans treated through VA health care systems (Yano et al., 2006). In addition, 22% of women veterans screened positive for MST (Kimerling et al., 2007) and an overwhelming majority (greater than 70%) of women veterans have described chronic and systemic problems with sexual harassment; the percentage is expected to be higher for the subgroup of SGM female veterans.

Postdeployment Experience

Studies conducted among veterans indicate that many veterans experience some adjustment problems and significant levels of violence, isolation, homelessness, mental illness and involvement with the criminal justice system postdeployment (Figley, 1978; Fontana & Rosenheck, 2005). Readjustment research from the Vietnam War provides a framework in which to explore the adjustment experience of SGM older veterans. Kulka et al. (1990) conducted the most rigorous and comprehensive study on the readjustment experience of Vietnam veterans (NVVRS) and found that combat exposure was more often linked to readjustment problems. In particular, Kulka et al. (1990) identified those with wartime stressors (deployed to Vietnam) to have higher divorce rates, more marital and relational problems, difficulty maintaining parental roles, and higher levels of family discord. Kulka et al. (1990) also noted in the NVVRS that deployed women veterans experienced more readjustment problems than nondeployed Vietnam Era female veterans. Studies conducted after the Persian Gulf War compared male and female veterans and found women veterans were more likely to report symptoms of distress (PTSD, anxiety, depression). Older OIF/OEF veterans may also experience significant distress as they age.

Homelessness

Homelessness continues to be a serious problem for 50,000 veterans as estimated during a recent point-in-time count of veterans in 2014. Homeless veterans have served in every conflict since World War II and almost 50% served during the Vietnam Era and are over the age of 50. In the United States, approximately 12% of the adult homeless population are veterans who are predominantly male, single, and live in cities, while a majority suffer from mental and physical disorders such as substance abuse or other co-occurring mental disorders. According to the National Alliance to End Homelessness (NAEH) factsheet on veteran homelessness (April, 2015), 40% of all homeless veterans are African American or Hispanic, even though they account for less than 10% of the veteran population. Aging SGM veterans struggle with less social support, lower socioeconomic status, and lower employment status relative to their heterosexual veteran peers. Food and housing insecurities as a veteran ages have the potential of compounding other health disparities and may lead to more deleterious outcomes. The NAEH (April, 2015) estimates approximately 1.5 million veterans suffer from food and housing insecurity and are at risk for homelessness as a result of poverty and substandard housing options. Although the VA continues to provide resources and advance programs for homeless veterans, many of these may be undesirable for SGM aging veterans. The marginal resources of community agencies caused by dwindling budgets and increased needs coupled with the unique needs of aging SGM veterans creates a perfect storm of unintended consequences and inadequate service provision.

BEST PRACTICES AND FUTURE DIRECTIONS

Health care professionals are in a unique and vital position to help aging SGM veterans with their service needs, supportive housing, and employment opportunities because they work in varied environments, providing services at multiple levels. Although the VHA is the largest health care employer in the nation, and VHA services have increased, current research estimates that the majority of veterans including aging SGM veterans do not utilize the VHA (Yano et al., 2011; Haskell et al., 2011). Therefore, it is paramount for community-based health professionals to recognize the needs of the "silent minority" group of veterans and become knowledgable about and offer in-service training on the needs and experiences of aging SGM veterans and their families. Encouraging and increasing the numbers of health care providers committed to the physical, mental, and environmental health care needs of aging veterans, and specifically SGM veterans, is essential. Health educators must provide an integrative curriculum that highlights the positive features of working with the aging population. Additionally, it is paramount that the needs of SGM aging veterans are not overlooked. Helping to create meaningful supportive services is just one way all service providers can make a profound difference in the lives of those who have given so much of themselves in the service of others.

The importance of further study on SGM aging veterans cannot be overstated. SGM aging veterans have unique health care needs and significant health disparities compared to both their military peers and civilians. Utilizing community-based research data will expand awareness of all the issues and barriers to care among this vulnerable population. Program development and service delivery will be enhanced by continuing to explore the health care needs.

The physical and mental health care needs of aging SGM veterans is an important area for professional health education, research, program development, and service provision. Without committed, progressive, and emphatic health care providers at all levels, the needs of this important aging cohort will continue to be overlooked. Quantitative and qualitative research that focuses on community-based SGM aging veterans is an important step in that direction. Program development that integrates the special needs of aging veterans, while providing incentives to early career health professionals to work in the field of geriatrics is essential. Finally, health care education needs to take an aggressive and activist role in challenging and addressing the stigma of working with older adults, and in particular aging SGM veterans.

REFERENCES

Ailshire, J. A., & Crimmins, E. M. (2011). Psychosocial factors associated with longevity in the United States: Age differences between the old and oldest-old in the health and retirement study. *Journal of Aging Research*, *2011*, 1–10.

Basham, K. (2008). Homecoming as safe haven or the new front: Attachment and detachment in military couples. *Clinical Social Work Journal*, *36*(1), 83–96.

Blosnich, J., Bossarte, R., Silver, E., & Silenzio, V. (2013). Health care utilization and health indicators among a national sample of U.S. Veterans in same-sex partnerships. *Military Medicine*, *178*(2), 207–212.

Blosnich, J., Foynes, M. M., & Shipherd, J. C. (2013). Health disparities among sexual minority women veterans. *Journal of Women's Health*, *22*(7), 631–636.

Blosnich, J. R., Bossarte, R. M., & Silenzio, V. M. (2012). Suicidal ideation among sexual minority veterans: Results from the 2005–2010 Massachusetts Behavioral Risk Factor Surveillance Survey. *American Journal of Public Health*, *102*(S1), S44–S47.

Blosnich, J. R., & Silenzio, V. M. B. (2013). Physical health indicators among lesbian, gay, and bisexual U.S. veterans. *Annals of Epidemiology*, *23*, 448–451.

Booth, B. M., Davis, T. D., Cheney, A. M., Mengeling, M. A., Torner, J. C., & Sadler, A. G. (2012). Physical health status of female veterans: Contributions of sex partnership and in-military rape. *Psychosomatic Medicine*, *74*, 916–924.

Brennan-Ing, M., Seidel, L., Larson, B., & Karpiak, S. E. (2014). Social care networks and older LGBT adults: Challenges for the future. *Journal of Homosexuality*, *61*, 21–52.

Burks, D. J. (2011). Lesbian, gay, bisexual victimization in the military: An unintended consequence of "Don't ask, Don't tell"? *American Psychologist*, *66*(7), 604–613.

Cochran, B. N., Balsam, K., Flentje, A., Malte, C. A., & Simpson, T. (2013). Mental health characteristics of sexual minority veterans. *Journal of Homosexuality*, *60*, 419–435.

Cohen, S. & Syme, L. S. (1985). Issues in the study and application of social support. In S. Cohen & L. S. Syme (Eds.), *Social support and health* (pp. 3–20). New York, NY: Academic Press.

Cohen, L. H., Hettler, T. R., & Park, C. L. (1997). Social support, personality, and life stress adjustment. In G. R. Pierce, B. Lakey, I. G. Sarason, & B. R. Sarason (Eds.), *Sourcebook of social support and personality.* New York, NY: Plenum Press.

Cotten, S. R., & Skinner, K. M. (2000). Social support among women veterans. *Journal of Women and Aging, 12*(1), 39–62.

Defense Department Advisory Committee on Women in the Services. (2013). Report. DD-P&R (AR) 2535. Retrieved from http://dacowits.defense.gov/ReportsMeetings.aspx

Der-Martirosian, C., Cordasco, K. M., & Washington, D. L. (2013). Health-related quality of life and comorbidity among older women veterans in the United States. *Quality of Life Research*, *22*, 2749–2756.

Everett, J. E., Hall, J. C., & Hamilton-Mason, J. (2010). Everyday conflict and daily stressors: Coping response of Black women. *Journal of Women and Social Work, 25*(1), 30–42.

Figley, C. R. (1978). Psychological adjustment among Vietnam veterans: An overview of the research. In C. R. Figley (Ed.), *Stress disorders among Vietnam veterans: Theory, research, and treatment* (pp. 57–70). New York, NY: Brunner/Mazel.

Fontana, A., & Rosenheck, R. (2005). The role of war-zone trauma and PTSD in the etiology of antisocial behavior. *Journal of Nervous and Mental Disease, 193*(3, March), 203–209.

Fontana, A., Rosenheck, R., & Horvath, T. (1997). Social support and psychopathology in the war zone. *Journal of Nervous and Mental Disease, 185*(11), 675–681.

Frayne, S. M., Parker, V. A., Christiansen, C. L., Loveland, S., Seaver, M. R., Kazis, L. E., Skinner, K. M. (2006). Health status among 28,000 women veterans: The VA women's health program evaluation project. *Journal of General Internal Medicine, 21*(3), S40–S46.

Fredriksen-Goldsen, K. I., Emlet, C. A., Kim, H., Muraco, A., Erosheva, E. A., Goldsen, J., Hoy-Ellis, C. P. (2012). The physical and mental health of Lesbian, Gay Male, Bisexual (LGB) older adults: The role of key health indicators and risk and protective factors. *The Gerontologist*, *53*(4), 664–675.

Fredriksen-Goldsen, K. I., Kim, H., Shiu, C., Goldsen, J., & Emlet, C. A. (2014). Successful aging among LGBT older adults: Physical and mental health-related quality of life by age group. *The Gerontologist*, *55*(1), 154–168.

Gates, G. J. (2010). Lesbian, gay, and bisexual men and women in the U.S. military: Updated estimates. *The Williams Institute,* UCLA School of Law.

Gates, G. J., & Herman, J. L. (2014). *Transgender military service in the United States*. Los Angeles, CA: The Williams Institute, UCLA School of Law. Retrieved from http://williamsinstitute.law.ucla.edu/research/military-related/us-transgender-military-service/

Haskell, S. G., Mattocks, K., Goulet, J. L., Krebs, E. E., Skanderson, M., Leslie, D., et al. (2011). The burden of illness in the first year home: Do male and female VA users differ in health conditions and healthcare utilization. *Women's Health Issues, 21*(1), 92–97.

Herek, G. M. (2007). Confronting sexual stigma and prejudice: Theory and practice. *Journal of Social Issues*, *63*(4), 905–925.

House, J. S., & Kahn, R. L. (1985). Measures and concepts of social support. In S. Cohen & S. L. Syme (Eds.), *Social support and health* (pp. 83–108). New York, NY: Academic Press.

Institute of Medicine. (2011). *The health of lesbian, gay, bisexual, and transgender people: Building a foundation for better understanding*. Washington, DC: National Academy of Science Press.

Kimerling, R., Gima, K., Smith, M. W., Street, A., & Frayne, S. (2007). The Veterans health administration and military sexual trauma. *American Journal of Public Health, 97*(12), 2160–2166.

Kulka, R. A., Schlenger, W. E., Fairbank, J. A., Hough, R. L., Jordan, K., Marmar, C. R., et al. (1990). *Trauma and the Vietnam War generation: Report of the findings from the National Vietnam veteran's readjustment study*. New York, NY: Routledge.

Lehavot, K., Hoerster, K. D., Nelson, K. M., Jakupcak, M., & Simpson, T. L. (2012). Health indicators for military, veteran, and civilian women. *American Journal of Preventive Medicine, 42*(5), 473–480.

Lehavot, K., & Simpson, T. L. (2012). Incorporating lesbian and bisexual women into women veterans' health priorities. *Journal of General Internal Medicine*, *28*(2), S609–614.

Mankowski, M., Mattocks, K. M., Haskell, S., & Brandt, C. (2015). Social support throughout the deployment cycle for women veterans returning from Iraq and Afghanistan. *Social Work in Health Care, 54*(4), 287–306.

Mattocks, K. M., Haskell, S. G., Krebs, E. E., Justice, A. C., Yano, E. M., & Brandt, C. (2012). Women at war: Understanding how women veterans cope with combat and military sexual trauma. *Social Science and Medicine,* 1–9. http://dx.doi.org/10.1016/j.socscimed.2011.10.039

Mattocks, K. M., Kauth, M. R., Sandfort, T., Matza, A. R., Sullivan, J. C., & Shipherd, J. C. (2013a). Understanding health-care needs of sexual and gender minority veterans: How targeted research and policy can improve health. *LGBT Health*, *1*(1X), 1–8.

Mattocks, K. M., Sadler, A., Yano, E. M., Krebs, E. E., Zephyrin, L., Brandt, C., et al. (2013b). Sexual victimization, health status, and VA healthcare utilization among lesbian and bisexual OEF/OIF veterans. *Journal of General Internal Medicine, 28*(2), S604–608.

Meyer, I. H. (2003). Prejudice, social stress, and mental health in lesbian, gay, and bisexual populations: Conceptual issues and research evidence. *Psychological Bulletin, 129*(5), 674–697.

Moradi, B. (2009). Sexual orientation disclosure, concealment, harassment, and military cohesion: Perceptions of LGBT military veterans. *Military Psychology*, *21*, 513–533.

Moran, D. (2013). Leading the way in policy implementation: An examination of how the United States Marine Corps has managed the Don't Ask Don't Tell repeal. *Journal of Public Management and Social Policy, 19*(1), 81–90.

Mulhall, E. (2009). *Women warriors: Supporting she who has borne the battle*. Iraq Women's Veterans of America (IAVA). Washington, DC: US Department of Defense Issue Report. Retrieved from http://media.iava.org/IAVA_WomensReport_2009.pdf

National Alliance to End Homelessness. (2015). *Factsheet on veteran's homelessness*. Retrieved from http://www.endhomelessness.org/library/entry/fact-sheet-veteran-homelessness

National Defense Authorization Act, Pub. L. No. 103-160, 10 U.S.C. § 654, (1994).

Office of Disease Control and Health Prevention, National Center for Health Statistics. (2014). *Lesbian, gay, bisexual, and transgender health*. Retrieved from https://www.healthypeople.gov/2020/topics-objectives/topic/lesbian-gay-bisexual-and-transgender-health

Sanders, J. B., Comijs, H. C., Bremmer, M. A., Deeg, D. J. H., & Beekman, A. T. F. (2015). A 13-year prospective cohort study on the effects of aging and frailty on the depression–pain relationship in older adults. *International Journal of Geriatric Psychiatry*, *30*(7), 751–757.

Simpson, T. L., Balsam, K. F., Cochran, B. N., Lehavot, K., & Gold, S. D. (2013). Veterans Administration Health Care utilization among sexual minority veterans. *Psychological Services*, *10*(2), 223–232.

Stuart, J. A., Murray, K. M., Ursano, R. J., & Wright, K. M. (2002). The Department of Defense Persian gulf war registry year 2000: An examination of veterans' health status. *Military Medicine, 167*, 121–128.

The Joint Commission on Veterans Affairs. (2011). *Advancing effective communication, cultural competence, and patient-and family-centered care for the lesbian, gay, bisexual, and transgender (LGBT) community: A field guide*. Retrieved from http://www.jointcommission.org/assets/1/18/LGBTFieldGuide.pdf

Thoits, P. A. (1995a). Identity-relevant events and psychological symptoms: A cautionary tale. *Journal of Health and Social Behavior, 36*, 72–82.

Thoits, P. A. (1995b). Stress, coping, and social support processes: Where are we? What's next? *Journal of Health and Social Behavior, Extra Issue*, 53–76.

Tucker, M. A., & Kelley, M. L. (2009). Social support and life stress as related to the psychological distress of single enlisted Navy mothers. *Military Psychology, 21*(Suppl. 2), 82–97.

Unutzer, J. (2007). Late-life depression. *New England Journal of Medicine, 357*, 2269–2276.

U.S. Census Bureau. (2012). *Today, there are 9.4 million veterans ages 65 and over* (U.S. Census, 2012). Retrieved from http://www.agingstats.gov/main_site/data/2012_documents/population.aspx

U.S. Department of Veterans Affairs. (2015). *National Center for Veterans Analysis and Statistics*. Retrieved from http://www1.va.gov/vetdata

U.S. Veterans Affairs, Veterans Health Administration. (2013). *VHA Directive 2013-003: Providing health care for Transgender and Intersex Veterans, 2013*. Retrieved from www.va.gov/vhapublications/ViewPublication.asp?pub_ID=2863

Ware, J. E. (1993). *SF-36 health survey: Manual and interpretation guide*. Boston, MA: The Health Institute, New England Medical Center.

Wills, T. A. (1985). Supportive functions of interpersonal relationships. In S. Cohen & L. S. Syme (Eds.), *Social Support and Health,* (pp. 61–78) New York, NY: Academic Press.

Yano, E. M., Bastian, L. A., Bean-Mayberry, B., Eisen, S., Frayne, S., Hayes, P., et al. (2011). Using research to transform care for women veterans: Advancing the research agenda and enhancing research-clinical relationships. *Women's Health Issues, 21*(4S), S73–S83.

Yano, E. M., Bastian, L. A., Frayne, S. M., Howell, A. L., Lipson, L. R., McGlynn, G., et al. (2006). Toward a VA women's health research agenda: Setting evidence-based priorities to improve the health and health care of women veterans. *Journal of General Internal Medicine, 21*(3), S93–S101.

CHAPTER 9

LGBT Aging in the Rural Context

Sandra S. Butler

ABSTRACT

This chapter examines the experiences of lesbian, gay, bisexual, and transgender (LGBT) older adults living in rural regions of the United States. It begins by reviewing the two concepts of rural and nonmetropolitan, how they differ from one another, and the difficulty in comparing studies of rural populations because of the resulting ambiguity in definition between the two. Despite these challenges, there exists a broad literature on rural populations, and the chapter reviews three aspects of rural communities: the conditions and status of older rural adults; what is known about the lives of rural LGBT adults of all ages; and finally, the specific issues and concerns of rural LGBT older adults. In general, nonmetropolitan areas are more conservative and homophobic than metropolitan centers, causing many LGBT individuals in these regions of the country to remain closeted in some aspects of their lives. Moreover, the low population density in rural areas leads to far fewer opportunities for LGBT-specific social gatherings. These difficulties are compounded for older, rural LGBT adults who may have less access to transportation, less comfort with online social networking, and may be more fearful of disclosure due to growing up and coming out prior to gay liberation and the development of more progressive policies. The chapter concludes with best practices for practitioners working with rural, LGBT older adults and future trends for this particular population, given the recent dramatic changes in policy related to same-sex marriage and the ubiquity of high-speed Internet enhancing opportunities for connecting online.

http://dx.doi.org/10.1891/0198-8794.37.127

INTRODUCTION

Seventy-five percent of the United States is considered rural, home to over 50 million people (Johnson, 2012). While most research on lesbian, gay, bisexual, and transgender (LGBT) adults has been drawn from urban samples, we know from recent census data including information on same-sex couples that, gay men and lesbian women exist in all 50 states (Lee & Quam, 2013). Moreover, data from the 2000 Census indicated that 15% of the nearly 600,000 households headed by same-sex couples were located outside metropolitan areas (Lee & Quam, 2013); this represents over 88,000 gay and lesbian families (Grant, 2009), many of which may include older adults, or if not, may be families who choose to age in these rural settings.

For many individuals, rural living is seen as safer, healthier, and less stressful than life in the city (Watkins & Jacoby, 2007). Moreover, despite higher rates of poverty and a paucity of health and social service resources, rural America is still nostalgically referred to as the "heartland" (Lindhorst, 1997). But how does a stigmatized, often marginalized, sexual minority experience this rural idyll? Although there are significant regional differences, rural Americans are, in general, more conservative and more religious than their urban counterparts. They are more likely to identify as born-again Christians and "by extension are likely to embrace the traditional views associated with Christian exclusion" (Dillon & Savage, 2006, p. 9), such as opposition to abortion and same-sex marriage. So while the rural idyll may exist for some, Watkins and Jacoby (2007) underscore that rural culture "will always define those who belong and those who are different. It will serve to exclude those perceived to transgress the values of the idyll" (p. 861).

This chapter explores how being different impacts the lives of older LGBT individuals who reside in nonmetropolitan regions of the United States. The first section reviews how the terms rural and nonmetropolitan are defined by official sources and in the literature. This is followed by a brief review of the literature on rural aging. The next section summarizes what is generally known about the lives of LGBT individuals living in rural regions of the country, which is followed by a section reviewing the literature specifically addressing the experiences of older LGBT adults in rural areas. The chapter concludes by considering how recent policy changes and trends might impact the future lives and experiences of rural LGBT older adults.

DEFINING WHAT IS MEANT BY RURAL

There is not one clear definition of rural, making comparisons among studies on rural populations difficult and population estimates variable. Two recent books on rural aging devote considerable attention in their introductory chapters to these differing definitions, the content of which informs the following discussion (Goins & Krout, 2006; Krout & Hash, 2015). The two most commonly used definitions are those used by the U.S. Office of Management and Budget (OMB) and the U.S. Census Bureau (Goins & Krout, 2006; Krout & Hash, 2015). The OMB uses the terms metropolitan and nonmetropolitan, with counties serving as the unit of analysis. A Metropolitan Statistical Area (MSA) is defined as having one or more cities with 50,000 residents, an urbanized area, and total MSA of 100,000, or one or more outlying counties with close economic and social integration with a core metropolitan area (Goins & Krout, 2006; Krout & Hash, 2015). Nonmetropolitan Statistical Areas—what we often call rural—are all those counties that do not meet the metropolitan criteria and may include small cities, towns, and vast open space. This complicated definition was revised in 2000 by the OMB to identify Core Based Statistical Areas (CBSA)—or urban—and Outside CBSAs—or rural. The revision reduced the nonmetropolitan population from 55 to 49 million in 2000 (Goins & Krout, 2006).

The U.S. Census Bureau definition of urban and rural is less complex, but also less commonly used by federal agencies (Krout & Hash, 2015). Urban areas are defined as all incorporated cities or towns with populations of at least 2,500, with the rural designation being the residual category that includes all other regions. To complicate matters further, the definition of metropolitan does not perfectly match the definition of urban, nor does nonmetropolitan always mean rural. For example, in the 2000 U.S. Census, 11% of the population was categorized as both rural and metropolitan, while 7% was classified as urban and non metropolitan (Goins & Krout, 2006). Moreover, the general categories describe widely different regions. The urban category includes both large cities and rather small towns, while the rural category includes villages of up to 2,500 inhabitants and vast frontier land (Krout & Hash, 2015).

Clearly defining what we mean by rural is not an exact science. The studies reviewed in this chapter reflect that ambiguity, with rural being a rather amorphous concept. Despite the lack of precision, many have studied what it means to age in a rural context, some have examined the experience of living as a sexual minority outside metropolitan regions, and a few have combined these areas of scholarship to examine the lives of older LGBT rural adults.

AGING IN A RURAL CONTEXT

Just as the population of the entire United States—and for that matter the entire world—is aging, so too are populations in rural regions of the country. Rural areas have a disproportionate share of the country's older adults. Fifteen percent of the population in nonmetropolitan areas is composed of individuals 65 years of age and older, while the concentration is only 12% in metropolitan regions. Furthermore, the more sparsely populated an area, the older its population (Glasgow & Berry, 2013). Nationally, one in five older adults live rurally (Krout & Hash, 2015).

While there has been increasing attention in the field of gerontology to the study of rural aging, with a number of books devoted to the topic, on balance, both scholars and policy makers tend to neglect the particular experiences and challenges faced by rural older adults (Krout & Hash, 2015). Compared to their urban counterparts, rural elders tend to be less educated, have lower incomes, and have less adequate housing (Butler & Kaye, 2003; Goins & Krout, 2006). They also tend to have higher rates of chronic diseases, including obesity (Morton & Weng, 2013) and more acute health conditions. They also are more likely to rate their health as poor than are metropolitan elders (Butler & Kaye, 2003; Goins & Krout, 2006; Van Nostrand, 1993). Moreover, studies indicate that rural older adults have more mental health problems but seek treatment less often than urban older adults, reflecting, in part, the dearth of treatment options available in rural regions (Maiden, 2003). Furthermore, rural adults are more dependent on their private vehicles, given a lack of transportation alternatives, a situation that becomes increasingly challenging with advancing age. Compounding this situation is the distance to social and health services that rural residents must travel, given the smaller number and narrow range of services available (Butler & Kaye, 2003; Goins & Krout, 2006; Hash, Wells, & Spencer, 2015; Glasgow & Berry, 2013; Morton & Weng, 2013).

Despite these challenges, older adults in rural parts of the country do not necessarily see themselves as worse off than their urban counterparts, with several factors placing rural elders at an advantage over older adults in cities: more involvement in community activities, receipt of more support from local organizations, less fear of crime, and less abrupt retirement (Krout, 1988). Kivett (1988) also found perceived well-being of rural older adults to be equal to or greater than that of urban older adults, due in part to their long-standing reciprocal relationships with neighbors, a sense of uncrowdedness, and the sense that friends were more important than money. Supporting the salience of uncrowdedness, Butler and Cohen (2010) found that nature or "aesthetic capital" emerged as an important contributing concept to the perceived well-being of rural elders. Given these contributors to rural well-being, it is perhaps not surprising that Krout (1988) found life satisfaction for older adults increases as community size decreases.

Despite these generalities about rural aging, it is important to remember that there exists tremendous diversity within and between rural regions of the country. Not only do the rural regions themselves differ (e.g., the open spaces of ranchland in Wyoming compared to the rolling hills and small villages of Vermont) but so too does the composition of the population in terms of race, culture, religion, economic livelihood, and for the purposes of this chapter, sexual identity and orientation.

SEXUAL MINORITIES IN RURAL AMERICA

As stated earlier, rural regions are far from homogeneous. Nonetheless, data from the nationally representative General Social Survey indicate that rural Americans are more likely than their urban counterparts to attend church and to identify as born-again Christians. Not surprisingly, they are also more likely to oppose abortion and same-sex relations (Dillon & Savage, 2006). Given the generally more conservative context, what is it like for LGBT individuals to grow up, live, work, bring up their families, and have social lives in nonmetropolitan parts of the country?

This question has been investigated through a number of small sample studies spanning the past three decades. It should be noted that most studies focus on gay and lesbian populations, occasionally mentioning bisexual individuals, and very rarely, and only recently, have the experiences of transgender adults been included. As early as 1980, Moses and Buchner published an article titled "The Special Problem of Rural Gay Clients," cited in D'Augelli and Hart (1987), which described how gay individuals and lifestyles would be seen as completely contradictory to rural values of marriage, traditional family living, appropriate gender roles, and religious morality. D'Augelli and Hart (1987) underscore that in the 1980s, what was known about rural LGBT individuals was based on isolated incidents, anecdotal reports, and speculation. They submitted that nongay professionals were not knowledgeable about nor actively affirming of their gay clients and that gay helping professionals were generally cautious about coming out due to fear of loss of jobs and respect. This early article exposed the issue that has been reiterated in the three decades since its publication: the difficulty of finding gay community in often isolated rural locations.

Since these earlier descriptions of the experiences of sexual minorities in rural America, numerous small empirical studies have increased our knowledge of the experiences of LGBT individuals in various rural regions of the country. In the 1990s, Cody and Welch (1997) examined the life experiences and coping styles of 20 gay men living in nonmetropolitan northern New England and identified both positive and negative aspects of rural living. Included among the positive aspects were the simplicity and comfort of living in a small town, the beauty of their surroundings, and the proximity of outdoor recreational activities. Some also believed rural environments led to strong bonds with partners and other gay male friends. However, most study participants also said rural life was isolating, with few opportunities to meet other gay men. At the time of the study, the loss of so many friends to the AIDS epidemic was strongly felt by study participants, exacerbating the sense of aloneness. Some feared losing the few friendships they had if they were to come out, so they traveled to cities to find gay community.

The literature about rural gay life in the 1990s often mentioned the communal rural living or "land bands" created by groups of feminist lesbians between 1965 and 1985. Lindhorst (1997) and Bell and Valentine (1995) described these intentional women's communities, the latter quoting a full-length 1985 book on the subject by Joyce Cheney called *Lesbian Land*. For example, one woman from this back to the land movement said:

> The city has a way of making you feel trapped . . . when I did come here and the vision began to unfold even more, I knew this was the place and I had not chosen it, but She, my Mother Earth, had chosen me to come here. (quoted from Cheney [1985] in Bell & Valentine, 1995, pp. 118–119)

Bell and Valentine (1995), although describing "queer country" in the United Kingdom, underscore issues and themes common to the U.S. experience. One finding, which may still be salient for older gay and lesbian rural adults, is that some rural LG individuals deny the label of homosexual, let alone gay. Moreover, "due to the intense heteronormativity pressures of rural life" (p. 116), many are married, though do not necessarily identify as bisexual. Ultimately, similar to Cody and Welch (1997), Bell and Valentine (1995) describe the diversity of experience for rural gay men and lesbian women. The rural context is both a place of escape from the evils of the city for some, but for others, it offers only isolation and loathing.

The study of the LGBT experience in rural America has been further documented in the 21st century. Boulden (2001) examined the experiences of gay men in Wyoming through a small qualitative study ($n = 8$) and found that participants were very vigilant about how and when they came out or were "visibly gay." Others said if they were too out, their gay friends would avoid them so as not to be associated with being gay. In general, Boulden (2001) submits that the heterosexism of the rural state leads to a "don't ask, don't tell" mentality that discourages gay people from being open. This invisibility allows myths and stereotypes to persist along with continued oppression, and potentially violence, against LGBT individuals. A larger study of gay men in Wyoming ($n = 39$) investigating the social/sexual environment of study participants was carried out to inform HIV/AIDS prevention programs (Williams, Bowen, & Horvath, 2005). Study participants reported social hostility and potential violence, leading to efforts to assimilate through self-regulation, and ultimately, resulting in social isolation. Another study of rural gay men examined the relationship between stigma and sexual risk behavior (Preston, D'Augelli, Kassab, & Starks, 2007). Based on a self-administered questionnaire of men (n = 414) who have sex with men in rural Pennsylvania, the study revealed that stigma experienced in rural communities was related to sexual risk taking, which served as a coping mechanism against the daily stress caused by intolerance.

Using a focus group of 10 nonmetropolitan lesbian women, McCarthy (2000) explored the challenges of sustaining a lesbian identity in a rural setting. She found that though her study participants initially felt very isolated, small networks of lesbian friends helped them maintain a sense of lesbian identity. As one participant said, "You just don't feel like you're a poppy trying to blend in a wheat field when you have a community" (as quoted in McCarthy, 2000, p. 91). Another participant described the lack of information she had coming out at age 20 in the small town where she grew up:

> I think around here, a lot of people don't know anything about being gay, especially if you're gay yourself but haven't come out yet. You don't know anything about it, because it is not in your face at all. You don't see any of it, you don't hear about it. Nobody knows anything about it. (as quoted in McCarthy, 2000, p. 90)

More recently, the *Journal of Lesbian Studies* devoted a special issue to the experiences of rural lesbians. Puckett, Horne, Levitt, and Reeves (2011) compared the experience of rural and urban lesbian mothers based on a sample of 414 mothers in same-sex relationships. Rural lesbian mothers reported higher rates of discrimination from both strangers and human service professionals than did their urban counterparts. Furthermore, neighbors and parents of the children's classmates were less likely to know of the family's lesbian status, underscoring the invisibility documented in many previous studies of rural-dwelling gays and lesbians. In this same journal issue, Hastings and Hoovery-Thompson (2011) described the heightened stigma, potential isolation, and conservative climate faced by rural lesbians and the role of psychotherapists to help lesbian clients deal with these unique challenges.

Otis (2008) addresses the difficulties in conducting empirical research with rural lesbian and gay people, contributing to the dearth of studies with larger and/or representative samples. Accessing samples and maintaining confidentiality can be particularly challenging in nonmetropolitan settings that lack visible gay organizations and communities. Oswald and Culton (2003) obtained one of the largest samples of nonmetropolitan LGBT individuals (n = 527) for their examination of rural gay life. They distributed surveys through organizations and networks in 38 rural Illinois counties, collecting data through open-ended questions on best and worst aspects of rural life. Respondents reported that the existing LGBT community was fragmented and closeted. For example, one man wrote about "being shunned by closet–cases who fear association" and another respondent noted "a whole underground community exists in this area but none of them will associate with me because I am out of the closet" (as quoted in Oswald & Culton, 2003, p. 75). Respondents reported dealing with the intolerance they faced through disclosure management, resulting in the solidification of friendships and family relationships and carving out niches of support in an otherwise conservative climate.

After the murder of Matthew Shepard, a gay young man in Wyoming, in 1998, Leedy and Connolly (2008) surveyed lesbian, gay, and bisexual individuals in that rural state (n = 87) about their community ties, level of disclosure, and discrimination. While most respondents reported some ties with LGB individuals within their communities, high levels of discrimination were also reported. For example, one man said, "When I came out, I was living in a town of 250 and those who knew me well were OK with it, those who didn't totally shunned me" (as quoted in Leedy & Connolly, 2008, p. 25). A study out of Australia (Gottschalk, 2007) documents similar issues for rural gay men and lesbians as those experienced in the United States: lack of anonymity, smaller communities, and fewer supportive services. Stigma reached severe levels in some cases as described by one woman: "The rural community I was living in held a town meeting where it was decided to get rid of the undesirables" (as quoted in Gottschalk, 2007, p. 41).

Several articles published since 2000 have looked specifically at homophobia and stigma in rural America. For example, a study of college students (n = 123) from Kentucky examined levels of homophobia as measured through comfort with gay men and lesbian women in public settings (Eldridge, Mack, & Swank, 2006). At the bivariate level, students from rural backgrounds reported more discomfort with gay individuals than students from more urban backgrounds, though this lost significance at the multivariate level. Snively, Kreuger, Stretch, Watt, and Chadha (2004) examined levels of homophobia among social work students from two Midwestern schools. Rural respondents were more homophobic than urban respondents and were also less likely to support equal rights for LGB individuals. Given that social workers form a central part of social service networks in rural areas, these findings reflect a disturbing situation for rural LGBT individuals.

Two articles by Willging, Salvador, and Kano (2006a, 2006b) examined the status of mental health care of LGBT adults in rural New Mexico. Ethnographic interviews with 20 rural providers (2006a) uncovered a lack of education about LGBT mental health issues and significant levels of homophobia. A second study (2006b) involved interviews with 36 rural LGBT individuals regarding help-seeking behavior. Participants indicated a distrust of the few professional options available and examples of inappropriate care were reported. The authors submit that rural LGBT individuals are often "pragmatic health consumers, strategically remaining silent about their sexuality and relying on family ties to access secular and sacred resources in rural areas" (p. 874). While there is a relatively substantial body of literature on the experiences of LGB, and sometimes T, individuals in rural areas of the country, which has increased significantly since the turn of the century, the experiences of older LGBT adults have been less fully explored.

OLDER LGBT ADULTS IN RURAL AREAS

The current older cohort of LGBT adults lived through an era of nonacceptance, legal condemnation, violence, and fear quite different from the experiences of younger adults living in the current era. Thus, examining the specific experiences and needs of older LGBT adults in rural regions of the country is important and, to date, rarely done.

An early study on this topic examined the perceptions and experiences of 21 late middle-aged and older lesbians living in rural Maine (Butler & Hope, 1999). Study participants raised concerns about health care access due to both their low incomes and rural residence, but also noted the presence of sensitive health care professionals—some of whom were lesbians known to them—in rural practices and hospitals. Fears related to potential homophobia should they need long-term care were also expressed. Comerford, Henson-Stroud, Sionainn, and Wheeler (2004) also explored the experiences of late middle-aged and older lesbians in rural New England. Similarly, this qualitative study exposed the importance of lesbian community to meeting the social and emotional support needs of study participants, something the authors noted might be harder to access as the study participants grew older and became less mobile. While heterosexual neighbors were enlisted to help with living-related tasks, they tended not to provide emotional support. A recently published case study on a single gay man who had lived his entire life in the rural Midwest presents a positive picture of aging as a rural gay man (Rowan, Giunta, Grudowski, & Anderson, 2013). The 80-year-old study participant had lost his life partner 16 years earlier but remained socially active, being in relatively good health and having rich social networks. While his rural context is not explicitly addressed, the theme of "disclosure management" of his sexual orientation reinforces findings of the literature described earlier for LGBT individuals in rural environments. A major finding of this study is that despite the very real challenges faced by LGBT individuals aging in nonmetropolitan areas of the country, life satisfaction is also possible.

King and Dabelko-Schoeny (2009) collected data from 20 LGB rural, middle-aged and older adults (aged 40+) through an online questionnaire with open-ended questions exploring health care utilization and support networks. Several themes that emerged were not specific to the LGBT population (e.g., transportation problems, distance to services, fear of medical debt), but others were, such as fear of disclosure of sexual orientation to health care providers, lack of benefits for same-sex partners, and isolation from gay communities. A secondary analysis of a nationwide sample of LGBT baby boomers (n = 1201) by Lee and Quam (2013) examined geographic differences among respondents. Differences were found between urban and rural respondents with respect to income, levels of "outness," and self-reported importance of LGBT identity, with rural respondents having, on average, lower levels on all three. Rural respondents also reported being more guarded about sexual orientation with their friends, family, neighbors, and coworkers. The authors caution aging-service providers in rural areas to be aware that LGBT elders may not disclose their sexual orientation and identity.

On the topic of providers of aging-related services, Knochel, Croghan, Moone, and Quam (2013) surveyed leaders of Area Agencies on Aging regarding their service to LGBT older adults. Urban-based agencies were more likely than agencies in rural regions to provide LGBT outreach and services, to believe in addressing LGBT issues, and to receive requests for assistance from self-identified LGBT older adults. An innovative project in the United Kingdom investigated the experiences of older lesbians and gay men living in rural regions of the country (Fenge & Jones, 2012; Fenge, Jones, & Read, 2010), exploring the notion of a rural idyll for groups who may be seen as different. A primary outcome of this project was a 30-minute fictional film, titled *Rufus Stone*. The film, which could be useful in training service providers in the rural United States as well, can be accessed online (http://vimeo.com/109360805).

In summary, a few key themes can be identified from existing literature on older LGBT adults living in rural areas. Rural contexts present challenges to aging in places with fewer social and health services and fewer transportation options. Incomes tend to be lower, on average, in rural areas, further compounding problems with access to social and health services as well as recreational activities. Moreover, nonmetropolitan regions tend to be more conservative and can be less welcoming to those who do not fit traditional roles and values. The fish bowl effect causes LGBT adults of all ages to manage their disclosure of sexual orientation and identity to prevent ostracism. This can lead to isolation, particularly as gay communities are often informal and small.

BEST PRACTICES

As discussed earlier, practitioners in rural regions, as compared to more urban environments of the country, may be dealing with communities with higher levels of homophobia and working with older LGBT clients who are both more cautious about disclosure of their sexual orientation and identity, and more isolated than their urban counterparts. Some authors have offered guidance to practitioners working with gay men and lesbian women in rural regions of the country. Smith (1998) focused on large system change suggesting that direct service practitioners in rural areas needed to be gay affirmative and push for opportunities to change rural communities and organizations that ostracize gays and lesbians based on stereotypes and homophobia. Lindhorst (1997) encouraged practitioners to educate themselves on how the social cohesion of communities can be difficult for sexual minorities who are seen as different and may fear exposure and ostracism and to be comfortable with their own sexual orientation "so they can celebrate and encourage the exploration of gay identity by their clients" (p. 8).

Foster (1997) reported on a small focus group of helping professionals working in rural regions of the Southeast to learn how negative public perceptions of gay men and lesbian women impacted their practice. All five members of the group said they were led to believe that "it was criminally wrong for people of the same sex to engage in intercourse and that it was an abomination against God" (p. 29). While these practitioners said they had matured and become more accepting with time, one participant said "We are all in recovery. We have been sold a bill of goods around sexual behavior that we all need to get over" (as quoted in Foster, 1997, p. 30). Foster encouraged practitioners in rural areas to work together and support one another to change perceptions of gays and lesbians, which can be difficult given the "fishbowl effect" of working in a rural context, where human service practitioners themselves can be ostracized if perceived as too challenging of accepted norms.

Ultimately, best practices for working with LGBT older adults in rural areas include:

- Understanding and supporting an individual's choice on identity management
- Normalizing LGBT identity by being comfortable and open about one's own sexual orientation and identity as a practitioner
- Creating LGBT-affirmative health and social service settings (e.g., through printed materials, intake forms, and office décor that includes older LGBT adults)
- Helping clients to find existing LGBT support networks (online or otherwise), particularly those that cater to older adults, as well as

working to create new opportunities for social connections among older LGBT adults

- Actively opposing and working against bias, homophobia, and judgment within agencies and the larger community
- Making visible and supporting pro-LGBT actions, attitudes, initiatives, and networks
- Advocating for civil rights for LGBT in states where they do not yet exist

FUTURE TRENDS AND DIRECTIONS

The literature reviewed in this chapter spans nearly 40 years, a time of great change for LGBT individuals in the United States. The speed of policy change is captured in the Lambda Legal YouTube video *From Criminals to Newlyweds* (available at lambdalegal.org) referring to two historic Supreme Court cases with an exact 10-year span separating them: *Lawrence v. Texas* on June 26, 2003 (overturning the Texas sodomy law) and *United States v. Windsor* on June 26, 2013 (overturning parts of the Defense of Marriage Act). And exactly 2 years later, on June 26, 2015, the Supreme Court again made history in *Obergefell v. Hodges*, ruling that the Constitution's guarantees of due process and equal protection under the law mean that states—even rural conservative states—can no longer ban same-sex marriage (Zodikoff & Butler, 2015).

As was stated earlier, rural regions in this country are far from monolithic. There is great diversity from region to region and the rural population as a whole has experienced increased diversity. Racial and ethnic minorities accounted for 83% of rural population growth between 2000 and 2010 (Johnson, 2012). Such change may well challenge the traditional values and culture in these rural areas.

Further, the Internet has revolutionized the ability of people to connect with one another. While some rural areas have less access to high-speed broadband width than urban areas, this is changing rapidly, giving formerly isolated LGBT individuals access to online gay communities. Admittedly, for some older LGBT adults, who may be less comfortable using computers or less attracted to online groups, this will have little impact. But, in the years ahead, the Internet has great potential to ease some aspects of rural isolation and even increase access to services through telehealth.

The national organization Services and Advocacy for GLBT Elders (SAGE) has a network of local affiliates around the country. (See sageusa.org/advocacy/sagenet.cfm for the list of affiliates.) Most of these affiliates exist in metropolitan counties, but in 2013, the rural state of Maine established the first statewide affiliate of SAGENet. SAGE Maine conducted a community needs assessment of LGBT older adults (Gugliucci, Weaver, Kimmel, Littlefield, Hennessey, & Hollander,

2012) and a study of practitioners to learn about the health environment of LGBT older adults in the state (Gugliucci & Weaver, 2014). These efforts have increased knowledge about and visibility of older LGBT individuals in Maine and have led to increased opportunities for social activities (see sagemaine.org for more information). Similar initiatives could be carried out in other rural parts of the country and likely will be in the coming years as LGBT baby boomers—many of whom came out post Stonewall and who will benefit from the recently more welcoming legal climate—move into their elder years.

Living rurally has both challenges and benefits for all older adults, including LGBT individuals. While still very real for the current cohort of LGBT elders, the issues of ostracism, ignorance, and isolation will hopefully lessen in the years ahead. But for that to happen, we must be vigilant in our efforts to push "for opportunities to change rural communities and organizations that resist gay people because of perceived negative stereotypes and ignorance" (Smith, 1998, p. 20). This can happen through coalition building within the LGBT community and also by building bridges to the wider community. We are in a time of exciting change that can benefit both current rural LGBT elders and the cohorts that follow.

REFERENCES

Bell, D., & Valentine, G. (1995). Queer country: Rural lesbian and gay lives. *Journal of Rural Studies, 11*(2), 113–122.

Boulden, W. T. (2001). Gay men living in a rural environment *Journal of Gay and Lesbian Social Services, 12*(3/4), 63–75.

Butler, S. S., & Cohen, A. L. (2010). The importance of nature in the well-being of rural elders. *Nature and Culture, 5*(2), 150–174.

Butler, S. S. & Hope, B. (1999). Health and well-being for late middle-aged and old lesbians in a rural area. *Journal of Gay and Lesbian Social Services, 9*(4), 27–46.

Butler, S. S., & Kaye, L. W. (2003). Rurality, aging and social work: Setting the context. In S. S. Butler & L. W. Kaye (Eds.), *Gerontological social work in small towns and rural communities* (pp. 3–18). New York, NY: Haworth Press.

Cody, P. J., & Welch, P. L. (1997). Rural gay men in northern New England. *Journal of Homosexuality, 33*(1), 51–67.

Comerford, S. A., Henson-Stroud, M. M., Sionainn, C., & Wheeler, E. (2004). Crone songs: Voices of lesbian elders on aging in a rural environment. *Affilia: Journal of Women and Social Work, 19*(4), 418–436.

D'Augelli, A. R., & Hart, M. M. (1987). Gay women, men, and families in rural settings: Toward the development of helping communities. *American Journal of Community Psychology, 15*(1), 79–93.

Dillon, M., & Savage, S. (2006). *Values and religion in rural America: Attitudes toward abortion and same-sex relations*. Carsey Institute, Issue Brief, no. 1. Retrieved from http://scholars.unh.edu/carsey/12

Eldridge, V. L., Mack, L., & Swank, E. (2006). Explaining comfort with homosexuality in rural America. *Journal of Homosexuality, 51*(2), 39–56.

Fenge, L., & Jones, K. (2012). Gay and pleasant land? Exploring sexuality, ageing and rurality in a multi-method, performative project. *British Journal of Social Work, 42*, 300–317.

Fenge, L., Jones, K., & Read, R. (2010). Connecting participatory methods in a study of older lesbian and gay citizens in rural areas. *International Institute for Qualitative Methodology, 9*(4), 320–333.

Foster, S. J. (1997). Rural lesbians and gays: Public perceptions, worker perceptions, and service delivery. In J. D. Smith & R. J. Mancoske (Eds.), *Rural gays and lesbians* (pp. 23–35). New York, NY: The Haworth Press.

Glasgow, N., & Berry, E. H. (2013). Introduction to rural aging in twenty-first century America. In N. Glasgow & E. H. Berry (Eds.), *Rural aging in 21st century America* (pp. 1–13). New York, NY: Springer Publishing.

Goins, R. T., & Krout, J. A. (2006). Introduction: Aging in rural America. In R. T. Goins & J. A. Krout (Eds.), *Service delivery to rural older adults* (pp. 3–20). New York, NY: Springer Publishing.

Gottschalk, L. H. (2007). Coping with stigma: Coming out and living as lesbians and gay men in regional and rural areas in the context of problems of rural confidentiality and social exclusion. *Rural Social Work and Community Practice, 12*(2), 31–46.

Grant, J. M. (2009). *Outing age: 2010: Public policy issues affecting gay, lesbian, bisexual, and transgender elders.* Washington, DC: Policy Institute, National Gay and Lesbian Task Force.

Gugliucci, M. R., & Weaver, S. A. (2014). *SAGE Maine survey report: Maine's health practitioners caring for older GLBT patients.* Retrieved from http://tamarackplace.com/SAGEHealthPractitionerSurveyReport.pdf

Gugliucci, M. R., Weaver, S. A., Kimmel, D. C., Littlefield, M., Hennessy, J., & Hollander, L. (2012). *Gay, lesbian, bisexual and transgender (GLBT) aging in Maine: A community needs assessment.* Retrieved from http://sagemaine.org/index.html

Hash, K. M., Wells, R., & Spencer, S. M. (2015). Who are rural elders? In K. M. Hash, E. Jurkowski, & J. A. Krout (Eds.), *Aging in rural places: Policies, programs, and professional practice* (pp. 23–41). New York, NY: Springer Publishing.

Hastings, S. L., & Hoover-Thompson, A. (2011). Effective support for lesbians in rural communities: The role of psychotherapy. *Journal of Lesbian Studies, 15*(2), 197–204.

Johnson, K. M. (2012). *Rural demographic change in the new century: Slower growth, increased diversity.* Carsey Institute, Issue Brief, no. 44. Retrieved from http://scholars.unh.edu/carsey/159

King, S., & Dabelko-Schoeny, H. (2009). "Quite frankly, I have doubts about remaining": Aging-in-place and health care access for rural midlife and older lesbian, gay and bisexual individuals. *Journal of LGBT Health Research, 5*, 10–21.

Kivett, V. R. (1988). Aging in a rural place: The elusive source of well-being. *Journal of Rural Studies, 4*(2), 125–132.

Knochel, K. A., Croghan, C. F., Moone, R. P., & Quam, J. K. (2013). Training, geography, and provision of aging services to lesbian, gay, bisexual and transgender older adults. *Journal of Gerontological Social Work, 55*(5), 426–443.

Krout, J. A. (1988). The elderly in rural environments. *Journal of Rural Studies, 4*(2), 103–114.

Krout, J. A., & Hash, K. M. (2015). What is rural? An introduction to aging in rural places. In K. M. Hash, E. Jurkowski, & J. A. Krout (Eds.), *Aging in rural places: Policies, programs, and professional practice* (pp. 3–22). New York, NY: Springer Publishing.

Lee, M. G., & Quam, J. K. (2013). Comparing supports for LGBT aging in rural versus urban areas. *Journal of Gerontological Social Work, 56*(2), 112–126.

Leedy, G., & Connolly, C. (2008). Out in the cowboy state. *Journal of Gay and Lesbian Social Services, 19*(1), 17–34.

Lindhorst, T. (1997). Lesbians and gay men in the country: Practice implications for rural social workers. In J. D. Smith & R. J. Mancoske (Eds.), *Rural gays and lesbians* (pp. 1–11). New York, NY: The Haworth Press.

Maiden, R. J. (2003). Mental health services for the rural aged. *Psychiatric Times, 20*(12), 41–46.

McCarthy, L. (2000). Poppies in a wheat field. *Journal of Homosexuality, 39*(1), 75–94.

Morton, L. W., & Weng, C. (2013). Health and healthcare among the rural aging. In N. Glasgow & E. H. Berry (Eds.), *Rural aging in 21st century America* (pp. 179–194). New York, NY: Springer Publishing.

Oswald, R. F., & Culton, L. S. (2003). Under the rainbow: Rural gay life and its relevance for family providers. *Family Relations, 52*, 72–79.

Otis, M. D. (2008). Issues in conducting empirical research with lesbian and gay people in rural settings. In W. Meezan & J. I. Martin (Eds.), *Handbook of research with lesbian, gay, bisexual and transgender populations* (pp. 280–299). Florence, KY: Routledge.

Preston, D. B., D'Augelli, A. R., Kassab, C. D., & Starks, M. T. (2007). The relationship of stigma to the sexual risk behavior of rural men who have sex with men. *AIDS Education and Prevention, 19*(3), 218–230.

Puckett, J. A., Horne, S. G., Levitt, H. M., & Reeves, T. (2011). Out in the country: Rural sexual minority mothers. *Journal of Lesbian Studies, 15*(2), 176–186.

Rowan, N. L., Glunta, N., Crudowski, E. S., & Anderson, K. A. (2013). Aging well and gay in rural America: A case study. *Journal of Gerontological Social Work, 56*, 185–200.

Smith, J. D. (1998). Working with larger systems: Rural lesbians and gays. In J. D. Smith & R. J. Mancoske (Eds.), *Rural gays and lesbians* (pp. 13–21). New York, NY: The Haworth Press.

Snively, C. A., Kreuger, L., Stretch, J. J., Watt, J. W., & Chadha, J. (2004). Understanding homophobia. *Journal of Gay and Lesbian Social Services, 17*(1), 59–81.

Van Nostrand, J. F. (1993). *Common beliefs about the rural elderly: What do national data tell us?* (National Center for Health Statistics, Vital Health Statistics, Vol. 3, No. 28). Washington, DC: Government Printing Office.

Watkins, F., & Jacoby, A. (2007). Is the rural idyll bad for your health? Stigma and exclusion in the English countryside. *Health and Place, 13,* 851–864.

Willging, C. E., Salvador, M., & Kano, M. (2006a). Unequal treatment: Mental health care for sexual and gender minority groups in a rural state. *Psychiatric Services, 57*(6), 867–870.

Willging, C. E., Salvador, M., & Kano, M. (2006b). Pragmatic help seeking: How sexual and gender minority groups access mental health care in a rural state. *Psychiatric Services, 57*(6), 871–874.

Williams, M. L., Bowen, A. M., & Horvath, K. J. (2005). The social/sexual environment of gay men residing in a rural frontier state: Implications for the development of HIV prevention programs. *The Journal of Rural Health, 21*(1), 48–55.

Zodikoff, B. D., & Butler, S. (2015). Social work with lesbian, gay, bisexual, and transgender older adults. In D. B. Kaplan & B. Berkman (Eds.), *Oxford handbook of social work in health and aging* (2nd ed., pp. 555–564). New York, NY: Oxford Press.

CHAPTER 10

Providing Health and Social Services to Older LGBT Adults

Andrea Daley, Judith A. MacDonnell, Shari Brotman,
Melissa St. Pierre, Jane Aronson, and Loralee Gillis

ABSTRACT

Little is known about the home care context for lesbian, gay, bisexual, and transgender (LGBT) older adults, most of whom, like the general older adult population, prefer to stay in their home and community for as long as possible. The very limited LGBT-focused home care literature available suggests that there are unique concerns about providing care in the home. In this chapter, access to affirmative home care services for LGBT older adults is located within the context of the LGBT health services access research literature. A program of research focused on identifying key access and equity indicators and associated prompts to assist organizations to provide high-quality, affirmative home care for these populations is described.

INTRODUCTION

In this chapter, issues of access and equity for lesbian, gay, bisexual, and transgender (LGBT) older adults are considered with a specific focus on home care in Ontario, Canada. First, an overview of the existing research literature on barriers to health services in general for older LGBT adults is provided focusing on lack of attention to their access to home care. Following this, an Ontario-based study of the home care access experiences of LGBT communities that deliberately

http://dx.doi.org/10.1891/0198-8794.37.143

included a subsample of participants aged 60 years and older is described. This is offered as an important program of research that seeks to extend considerations of barriers to health care services for LGBT older adults while underscoring the desire of these populations to age at home. The chapter concludes with an exploration of an access and equity (A & E) framework that was developed as a key component of the LGBT home care access research program in an effort to enhance access to high-quality, affirming care for LGBT older adults.

CURRENT RESEARCH

LGBT Health Services Access

In 2011, the American-based Institute of Medicine (IOM, 2011) pointed to the urgent need for improved equity and access to care for diverse groups of sexual and gender minorities. The gap in accessible care for older LGBT people has been well-documented (Brotman, Ferrer, Sussman, Ryan, & Richard, 2015; IOM, 2011) and poses a considerable risk to older LGBT people's health and well-being at a time when disability and chronic illness may require increased use of health services. Research has also indicated that the health issues facing older LGBT people are exacerbated by lifelong exposure to homophobic, biphobic, and transphobic discrimination and stigma (IOM, 2011). Despite this reality, older LGBT people remain considerably underrepresented in the mainstream health care system.

There has been increasing professional attention to the needs of older LGBT people in the health and social services literature (e.g., Fredriksen-Goldsen, Hoy-Ellis, Goldsen, Emlet, & Hooyman, 2014; Knochel, Croghan, Moone, & Quam, 2012; Leyva, Breshears, & Ringstad, 2014; Lim & Bernstein, 2012; Portz et al., 2014). A lengthy section of the IOM (2011) document on the current state of LGBT research was devoted to "Later Adulthood" in relation to LGBT populations. Two special journal issues on LGBT aging were published in 2014: the *Journal of Gerontological Social Work* (Erdley, Anklam, & Reardon, 2014; Fabbre, 2014; Fredriksen-Goldsen et al., 2014; McGovern, 2014; Portz et al., 2014; Rowan & Giunta, 2014; Siverskog, 2014; Sullivan, 2014) and the *Journal of Homosexuality*. The latter brought together contributions of community-based research to older LGBT health (Brennan-Ing, Seidel, Larson, & Karpiak, 2014; Brennan-Ing, Seidel, London, Cahill, & Karpiak, 2014; Croghan, Moone, & Olson, 2014; de Vries & Croghan, 2014; Gardner, de Vries, & Mockus, 2014; Morales, King, Hiler, Coopwood, & Wayland, 2014; Orel, 2014; Porter & Krinsky, 2014; Woody, 2014). A special issue of the *Clinical Gerontologist* on late life diversity offered an LGBT-focused article (Kimmel, 2014). The Registered Nurses Association of Ontario's (2007) position statement, *Respecting Sexual*

Orientation and Gender Identity identifies ageism and other social dynamics as affecting care for LGBT people. In 2015, the Gay and Lesbian Medical Association drew attention to the release of a position statement by the American Geriatrics Society (2015) on the care of LGBT older people. And finally, a recent award-winning documentary, *Gen Silent – The LGBT Aging Film* (Maddux, 2011), has raised the profile of the lived experiences of community-dwelling older LGBT people receiving home care and living in long-term care settings.

Much of the current literature on older LGBT people remains North American based (Gratwick, Jihanian, Holloway, Sanchez, & Sullivan, 2014; Harley & Teaster, 2016; IOM, 2011; Sears, 2013; Simone & Applebaum, 2011; Witten & Eyler, 2012). However, international contributions are increasing (Impact Report: LGBT Age Capacity Building Project, 2015; LGBT-Age-Audit-Tool, 2015; McCann, Sharek, Higgins, Sheerin, & Glacken, 2013; Neville & Henrickson, 2010; Peate, 2015; Stonewall, 2011; Westwood, King, Almack, Suen, & Bailey, 2015). In a Canadian context, research on/with LGBT older people has been emerging in relation to service delivery to meet the needs of diverse LGBT communities, for instance in long-term care settings generally, and most recently with a specific focus on trans aging (Aging Out, 2014; Brotman et al., 2015; City of Toronto Long-Term Care Homes and Services, 2008; Finkenauer, Sherratt, Marlow, & Brodey, 2012; Moore, 2009, Murray, Numer, Merritt, Gahagan, & Comber, 2011).

Concerns that LGBT older people often anticipate and face include multiple forms of discrimination from service agencies, leading to their avoidance of service access, a reality that is well-documented in the research literature. Gaps in professional education about LGBT older people and resulting experiences of heterosexism, homophobia, biphobia, transphobia, and cissexism[1] have been identified as key dynamics in the availability of and access to relevant programs and services (Brotman et al., 2015; Finkenauer et al., 2012; Fredriksen-Goldsen et al., 2014; Hardacker, Rubinstein, Hotton, & Houlberg, 2014; Hughes, Harold, & Boyer, 2011; Leyva et al., 2014; Lim & Bernstein, 2012; Portz et al., 2014; Siverskog, 2014). Consistently, research with health care providers suggests that many providers lack awareness of the holistic health issues of older LGBT people and that care providers in health and social service agencies often state that they have never cared for an older person who is LGBT-identified. Research with older LGBT people shows that such lack of provider awareness has consequences for accessing care that ranges from concerns about overt experiences of discrimination, stigma, and violence, to invisibility and erasure of identity to fears of disclosing their LGBT identities, which results in complete avoidance of care (Boggs et al., 2014; Bradford, 2013; Brotman et al., 2015; Gutman & Spencer, 2010; IOM, 2011; Kimmel, 2014; Moore, 2009; Siverskog,

2014; Witten & Eyler, 2012; Wright et al., 2014). This is evident across the health care spectrum including such services as mental health (Coon & Burleson, 2013; McGovern, 2014; Tinney et al., 2015); long-term care (Hovey, 2009; Moore, 2009; Schwinn & Dinkel, 2015); residential/assisted living (Aging Out, 2014; Neville & Henrickson, 2010); palliative and end-of-life care (Cartwright, Hughes, & Lienert, 2012; Rawlings, 2012); HIV services (Brennan-Ing, Seidel, London, et al., 2014; Vermette & Godin, 1996); and caregiver support (Brotman et al., 2007; Croghan et al., 2014).

Given the widespread unavailability and/or lack of expectation of affirming care, LGBT older adults' conscious decisions not to disclose their identities or identify people in their lives (such as same-sex partners) who are key to understanding their health can be understood as a discerningly self-protective strategy. The above body of literature on provider education at times speaks to strategies to remedy this gap with a focus on curriculum, workplace training in various sectors from long-term care to community programs, and identification of professional competencies. At times these activities are linked to the need for broader cultural competency initiatives at organizational and professional levels and the importance of structural change to foster health equity more comprehensively (Daley & MacDonnell, 2015).

The invisibility of diversity in LGBT research has implications for understanding these populations' needs and issues in relation to aging. For example, Lee and Brotman (2011) point to the reality that trans and bisexual people, people of color, and those with limited social privilege such as privileges of citizenship—for instance, LGBT im/migrants and refugees—are unlikely to be represented in current research (Fabbre, 2014; Siverskog, 2014). Yet, Canadian research suggests that racialization and language affect older people's access to care. Seven percent of Canadian seniors report a visible minority status, and half of newly immigrated seniors do not speak either English or French (Turcotte & Schellenberg, 2007).

It has been noted that incremental change in support of LGBT people generally has not benefitted all members of these communities. For example, racialized, poor, and immigrant LGBT people continue to struggle with limited access to many health, social care and community-based services, which have not been adapted to address interlocking forms of oppression (Van Sluytman & Torres, 2014). Such interlocking discrimination is an important consideration when examining older LGBT people's access to basic needs such as housing and senior-focused programs. For example, research has identified that LGBT older adults may encounter economic challenges that limit their ability to access specific programs (Chiplin, Chin, Dayton, Redman, & McIntyre, 2011) and benefit from health promotion strategies, an issue that is particularly salient for older lesbian and trans women who are often in a more financially vulnerable state than are men (Finkenauer et al., 2012; Fredriksen-Goldsen et al., 2013; Orel, 2014).

A recent systematic review of the literature on trans aging (Finkenauer et al., 2012), along with the extensive synthesis by the IOM (2011) highlights the unique issues that trans people face, while drawing attention to the diversity within these communities. For instance, these sources point to the particular needs of older people and lack of research that examines difference across the masculine through feminine spectrum of gender expression and identity. They also address social positioning in relation to ethnicity, poverty, employment status, and other differences that influences one's experience of aging and physical and mental health risk. In addition, trans people may face marginalization, discrimination, or lack of support from LGB communities (Witten & Eyler, 2012). As Brotman et al. (2015) note, for trans people, processes of gender expression and transition that can be the result of hormone treatment and/or surgical change manifest as bodily difference and/or incongruences between gender and name documentation in health systems. Such incongruences have implications for personal bodily care and privacy of health records and are especially relevant given the likelihood that the need for medical/health care will increase with age. "The self-protective strategy of non-disclosure may be impossible when receiving health care in these environments exposing transgender patients and clients to discrimination in the forms of rejection, ridicule, and hostility by staff and other residents" (Brotman et al., 2015, p. 122). Brotman et al. (2015) and Finkenauer et al. (2012) also consider the Canadian context of aging for trans people, pointing to concerns with research that subsumes trans health under LGBT research in general. As a consequence, there are risks of erasing the shifting nature of trans identities and associated transphobia that is layered over the dominant heteronormativity and cisnormativity embedded in health care interactions and systems of care.

Service utilization takes into account both formal and informal care. Although informal care is being addressed elsewhere in this volume, it is important for us to reiterate that older LGBT people may face unique challenges in this context, particularly if they are single or are lacking in social support from families of origin (Gabrielson, 2011a). For the many LGBT seniors who live alone (River, 2006; Rosenfeld, 2003; Stonewall, 2011), especially those who represent the oldest cohort of seniors and persons with a disability who have limited social networks (Brennan-Ing, Seidel, Larson, et al., 2014; Brotman, Ryan, & Cormier, 2003), the risk of isolation and thus negative health outcomes is exacerbated.

The reality of social isolation among LGBT older adults has been described as a function of social and historical discrimination, which resulted in more limited and ruptured interactions with biological family, the tremendous losses that occurred during the early years of the HIV/AIDS pandemic (Brotman et al., 2007), and the generalized ageism within queer communities that often leave older members excluded or invisible from community life (Brotman et al., 2003). However, although it is important to take social isolation into account, we must be careful not to overexaggerate the reality of loneliness among older LGBT adults (Brotman & Ferrer, 2015). The extent of the problem is often conflated by the lack of recognition of "fictive kin networks" made up of close friends (Muraco & Fredriksen-Goldsen, 2011). Alternative support systems, such as intergenerational friendship and community networks, reflect unique commitments within LGBT communities that are often unavailable to heterosexual older adults.[2] For example, informal activist community networks (such as those related to HIV/AIDS, lesbian feminist and trans-liberation movements) often come together to provide care and companionship to older members in need as a result of strong commitments to the ideals of "solidarity" or "sisterhood" built over several decades (Brennan-Ing, Seidel, Larson, et al., 2014; Gabrielson 2011a, 2011b; Sinding, 1999).

Generational differences within older LGBT communities have also influenced the visibility of those who challenge systems to make them more responsive. Morales et al. (2014) differentiate boomer (born 1946 through 1964) and silent (1925 through 1945) generations as a means of understanding differences in patterns of activism on issues of aging. These and other scholars have pointed to the reality that those with some vestiges of privilege (such as those representing financially secure, younger, White and/or gay male cohorts) are more likely to act as agents of change. For LGBT older adults, for whom the fears of losing services as a result of complaining are amplified, remaining silent and invisible is a key self-care strategy (Ward, River, & Fenge, 2008).

LGBT Home Care Access

Little is written about the home care context for older LGBT people, most of whom, like the general older adult population, prefer to stay in their home and community for as long as possible (Boggs et al., 2014; Bradford, 2013; Brotman et al., 2015; Ceci, Björnsdóttir, & Purkis, 2012; Geary & Schumacher, 2012; Graham, Ivey, & Neuhauser, 2009; Moore, 2009; National Gay and Lesbian Task Force, 2005; Van Wagenen, Driskell, & Bradford, 2013; Wright et al., 2014). In Ontario, over 50% of home care clients are over the age of 65 (Ontario Home Care Association, 2014).[3] The very limited LGBT-focused home care literature available suggests that there are unique concerns about providing care in the home (Daley & MacDonnell, 2015; Grigorovich, 2015a, 2015b, 2015c; Vermette & Godin, 1996).

Many LGBT older adults have expressed fears of having to hide books, pictures, and other 'indicators' of their sexual orientation in their own home to avoid discrimination by home care providers (Orel, 2014; Stein, Beckerman, & Sherman, 2010; Zodikoff, 2006). For those who experienced oppression in their young adult lives, "home" was often the only space in which they could live out their identities and relationships in safety and security. Requiring home care services often means jeopardizing this private space (Brotman et al., 2003). Previous research on fear of disclosure did not account for the particular realities of home care where the need for education and evaluation of home care providers is great. Unfortunately, low pay, lack of training, and high turnover of home care staff can often impede efforts to provide training (National Gay and Lesbian Task Force, 2005; River, 2006). This body of research on LGBT people may not accurately reflect issues facing the oldest old (80+) who are currently users of service but whose voices are rarely documented in research studies because they are difficult to reach or may be unable to participate due to ill health.

BEST PRACTICES: PROGRAMS, POLICIES, AND PROFESSIONAL PRACTICE

To date, there have been efforts to improve the health and social service experiences of LGBT older adults through queer organizing. In the U.S. context, for example, Services and Advocacy for GLBT Elders (SAGE) offers a broad range of services and programs aimed at improving the lives of older queer populations by reducing isolation and improving financial security, among other initiatives. In Canada, the Senior Pride Network focuses its advocacy work on expanding program and services for 50+. Changes in institutional family and next of kin policies (e.g., hospital, long-term care facilities) that recognize and affirm LGBT older adults, their partners, and support networks, albeit unevenly across national and international regions, also contribute to improving the lives of this population. Aligned with these and similar initiatives and the shift in service delivery to home care, we undertook several studies starting in 2009 as part of a research program that examines the landscape for understanding issues of access and equity specific to the home care context. This was undertaken in collaboration with Rainbow Health Ontario,[4] the Toronto Central Community Care Access Centre (CCAC),[5] and two community-based advisory committees. Through dialogue with our partners and our understanding that there was a gap in LGBT-related home care literature, one of our ultimate research goals was to create a tool that would enable home care provider agencies to assess their programs, policies, and practices in relation to equitable service access for LGBT populations, for example in relation to client intake forms, staff education, and other key issues informed by the literature. This section highlights the A & E framework developed as an outcome of this study, which can be used as an example of how best practices can be both implemented and evaluated across home care service sectors.

DISCURSIVE MAPPING OF HEALTH ACCESS AND EQUITY FRAMEWORKS

A synthesis of the "key indicators" literature on access and equity in health care organizations was conducted informed by a gender-based diversity analysis (Daley & MacDonnell, 2010, 2011).[6] A number of access and equity (A&E) frameworks were identified that often addressed the need for comprehensive program, policy, education, and leadership strategies to foster equitable care for LGBT people. Policy toolkits such as the LGBT Long-Term Care Toolkit (City of Toronto Long-Term Care Homes and Services, 2008) and the Seniors Mental Health Policy Lens Toolkit (McCourt, 2008) offer systematic and detailed strategies to create health promoting environments and programs for LGBT people and older people respectively. These tools include several key features such as attention to processes that promote the meaningful involvement of LGBT people/older adults reflecting their diversity and policies that impact the delivery of affirming services. No comparable home-care-specific A & E frameworks were identified through this process. In addition to these components of A & E frameworks, Daley and MacDonnell (2011) also identified a continuum of access and equity discourses that operated either implictly or explicitly, which served to frame initiatives at an ideological level, and which resulted in fostering or hindering access for LGBT people. These discourses can be understood as existing on a continuum from dominant discourses at one end to counterdiscourses on the other. Dominant discourses (such as those represented by multiculturalism or diversity) tended to water down issues to the level of individual or cultural problems and to the principle of equity as treating everyone the same. In these discourses, LGBT people risked becoming invisible or entirely absent. Counterdiscourses were more aligned with a rights-based perspective in which equitable access was viewed as a right and in which oppression was identified as a structural cause of inaccessibilty.

Second, findings from another study (MacDonnell & Daley, 2015)[7] that explored what it takes to create positive space were used to illustrate that in addition to addressing leadership, education/training, policies and programs, a key element of creating positive space was connected to engaging LGBT communities in organizational change and embedding a LGBT focus in the fabric of an organization. Finally, a study that explored the LGBT-specific training and education opportunities for home care service providers identified that personal support workers (PSWs), nurses, social workers, occupational therapists, and CCAC care coordinators had minimal and uneven access to LGBT-specific training and education, with unregulated providers (e.g., PSWs) being least likely to have these opportunities (Daley & MacDonnell, 2015). The lack of training and education opportunities for PSWs is a significant concern given the high frequency with which they interact with home care service users compared to other service provider groups. Overall, however, this key finding highlighted training/education as an important component to enhancing access to affirming care for LGBT older adults.

FUTURE DIRECTIONS: CONCEPTUALIZING ACCESS AND EQUITY

The development of an A & E framework has been integral to the goal of enhancing access to high-quality home care for LGBT people (Daley & MacDonnell, 2015; MacDonnell & Daley, 2015; Daley & MacDonnell, 2010). The framework incorporates six indicators of access to care for LGBT older adults to expose emerging gaps in research and strategies to address access to high-quality home care; leadership, environment, programs and services, community engagement, education and training, and policies (see Figure 10.1).

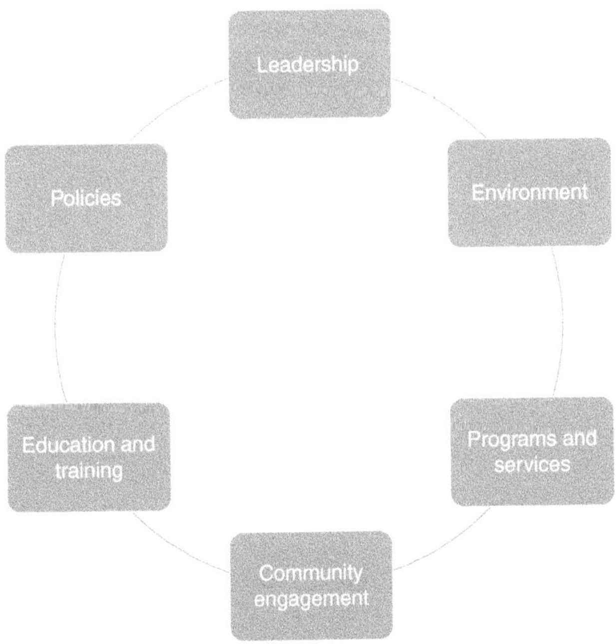

FIGURE 10.1 Home care access and equity framework.

Each component of the framework has associated evaluation prompts to assist organizations to consider programs, policies, and practices with respect to the provision of inclusive, affirming care for LGBT older adults (see Table 10.1). For example, prompts associated with community engagement ask whether and how home care organizations engage with LGBT people, and how community

TABLE 10.1
Home Care Access and Equity Framework Component Prompts

A & E Framework	Prompts
Community Engagement	Which LGBT people are involved in the community engagement process to ensure their diversity is represented?
	How are LGBT people engaged so that they can see themselves meaningfully represented in the agency and feel a sense of belonging?
Leadership	Are people at all levels of the organization involved in leadership opportunities including volunteers and allies associated with the organization?
	Are openly LGBT people in positions of leadership including 'out' senior management?
Environment	Are positive images of LGBT people included on organizational brochures, materials?
	How do staff use language to convey recognition, acceptance, and affirmation of LGBT people?
Policies	Are policies that address equity for LGBT service users and employees consistent across all programs?
	Do hiring practices include assessing diversity/LGBT competence? Do staff evaluation practices include assessing diversity/LGBT competency?
Education and Training	Who receives education and training within the agency?
	How does the organization advocate for resources for education/training for providers?
Programs and Services	How are LGBTQ people and/or staff involved in programming, agency processes (e.g., strategic planning)?
	How does the organization support a culture of disclosure for LGBT staff?

engagement strategies ensure the representation of diversity within LGBT communities. Prompts associated with training and education ask how diverse LGBT people are reflected and whether training occurs onsite or offsite of the agency, and how LGBT people are involved in the development of materials. (For a full description of the Access and Equity Framework and associated prompts please see Daley, MacDonnell, & St. Pierre, 2016).

The use of access and equity indicators and associated prompts holds the potential to create LGBT awareness in the context of home care organizations and open space for LGBT older adults to inform home care access and equity strategies. More specifically, the framework might be characterized as aligned with counterdiscourses or rather a rights-based perspective that could assist organizations to identify and change policies and practices that constitute structural causes of inaccessibilty for LGBT older adults (Daley & MacDonnell, 2011).

As indicated above, existing research documents barriers to health service access for LGBT older adults; however, it is limited in its attention to the unique context of home care. Contributing to this growing body of empirical evidence is research that focuses exclusively on the home care access experiences and realities among LGBT older adults (Daley & MacDonnell, 2015; MacDonnell & Daley, 2015). While the need for home care services is growing because of the aging population and increasing emphasis on keeping older people at home, little is known about the particular issues facing older LGBT people as they negotiate this type of care. Though LGBT community services are beginning to emerge, in the context of Canada, there is little funding for these services in the community, and they are only available in major cities such as Toronto or Vancouver. Most older LGBT adults requiring home care must receive it through the mainstream health service sector. This means that pressure must be put on these services to adapt to be inclusive and affirming in their care provision. Our project addresses this disjuncture by specifically looking at the design of access and equity as a framework to support LGBT inclusion within home care services in Ontario. An A & E framework (Daley & MacDonnell, 2010) helps home care organizations to consider inclusion through very specific indicators and prompts that can support inclusion. By building on the indicators to include LGBT older people's identities, expressions, and realities, we can further enhance service provision.

NOTES

1. Cissexism addresses discrimination for trans people, similar to what is termed "heterosexism" for lesbian, gay, bisexual, and queer (LGBQ) people. According to Grollman (2012), "Structural transphobic discrimination . . . occurs at the structural or societal level. This form of discrimination exists in laws, policies, and

macro-level values and practices that privilege cisgender people over transgender and gender non-conforming people. Structural transphobic discrimination is related to, or sometimes called, cissexism, the set of attitudes and behaviors which value and normalize cisgender people, while keeping transgender and gender non-conforming people invisible or treating them as inferior or deviant" (p. 1).

2. However, according to Brennan-Ing, Seidel, London, et al. (2014), "although this type of friend centered network has been typical of older GLBT adults…the same pattern is observed among heterosexual [Older People Living with HIV/AIDS] OPLWHA" (p. 169).

3. For an overview of the home care structure in Ontario, see Daley and MacDonnell (2015).

4. Rainbow Health Ontario is a province-wide program that works to improve the health and well-being of sexual and gender minority people, with a province-wide mandate.

5. The Toronto CCAC, located in central Toronto, is one of 14 CCACs in Ontario that coordinate home care services.

6. Funded by York University, Toronto, Ontario.

7. Funded by York University, Toronto, Ontario. We also conducted pilot research on the learning and training needs of diverse home care providers (Daley & MacDonnell, 2015), which identified the gap in LGBT-related education and training for home care providers with implications for interprofessional education.

REFERENCES

Aging Out. (2014, September). *Discussion paper. QCommunity. Vancouver, B.C.* Retrieved from http://qmunity.ca/wp-content/uploads/2015/03/AgingOut.pdf

American Geriatrics Society. (2015). American Geriatrics Society care of lesbian, gay, bisexual, and transgender older adults: Position statement. *Journal of the American Geriatrics Society, 9*(7), 423–426.

Boggs, J., Portz, J. D., Wright, L., King, D., Grimm, C., Retrum, J., et al. (2014). D3-4: The intersection of ageism and heterosexism: LGBT older adults' perspectives on aging-in-place. *Clinical Medicine and Research, 12*(1–2), 101.

Bradford, J. (2013, November). *Lifestyle preferences for older lesbians: Aging in place*. Paper presented at the 141st APHA Annual Meeting and Exposition, Los Angeles, CA.

Brennan-Ing, M., Seidel, L., Larson, B., & Karpiak, S. E. (2014). Social care networks and older LGBT adults: Challenges for the future. *Journal of Homosexuality, 61*(1), 21–52.

Brennan-Ing, M., Seidel, L., London, A. S., Cahill, S., & Karpiak, S. E. (2014). Service utilization among older adults with HIV: The joint association of sexual identity and gender. *Journal of Homosexuality, 61*(1), 166–196.

Brotman, S., & Ferrer, I. (2015). Diversity within family caregiving: Extending definitions of "who counts" to include marginalized communities. *Healthcare Papers, 15*(1), 47–53.

Brotman, S., Ferrer, I., Sussman, T., Ryan, B., & Richard, B. (2015). Access and equity in the design and delivery of health and social care to LGBTQ older adults: A Canadian perspective. In N. Orel & C. Fruhauf (Eds.), *Lesbian, gay, bisexual and transgender older adults and their families: Current research and clinical applications* (pp. 111–140). Washington, DC: American Psychological Association.

Brotman, S., Ryan, B., Collins, S., Chamberland, L., Cormier, R., Julien, D., et al. (2007). Coming out to care: Caregivers of gay and lesbian seniors in Canada. *The Gerontologist, 47*(4), 490–503.

Brotman, S., Ryan, B., & Cormier, R. (2003). The health and social service needs of gay and lesbian elders and their families in Canada. *The Gerontologist, 43*(2), 192–202.

Cartwright, C., Hughes, M., & Lienert, T. (2012). End-of-life care for gay, lesbian, bisexual and transgender people. *Culture, Health and Sexuality, 14*(5), 537–548.

Ceci, C., Björnsdóttir, K., & Purkis, M. E. (Eds.). (2012). *Perspectives on care at home for older people.* New York, NY: Routledge.

Chiplin, A. J., Jr., Chin, N., Dayton, K., Redman, D., & McIntyre, G. A. (2011). Older lesbian, gay, bisexual, and transgender individuals face special challenges in economic security and health care. *Clearinghouse Review: Journal of Poverty Law and Policy*, 44, 564–577.

City of Toronto Long-Term Care Homes and Services. (2008). *Diversity our strength: LGBT tool kit for creating lesbian, gay, bisexual and transgendered culturally competent care at Toronto long-term care homes and services.* Toronto, ON.

Coon, D. W., & Burleson, M. H. (2013). Working with gay, lesbian, bisexual, and transgender families. In G. Yeo & D. Gallagher-Thompson (Eds.), *Ethnicity and the dementias* (2nd ed., pp. 343–358). New York, NY: Routledge.

Croghan, C. F., Moone, R. P., & Olson, A. M. (2014). Friends, family, and caregiving among midlife and older lesbian, gay, bisexual, and transgender adults. *Journal of Homosexuality, 61*(1), 79–102.

Daley, A., & MacDonnell, J. A. (2015). 'That would have been beneficial': LGBTQ education for home care service providers. *Health and Social Care in the Community, 23*(3), 282–291.

Daley, A., MacDonnell, J. A., & St. Pierre, M. (2016, June). *LGBTTQI Communities and Home Care in Ontario: Project Report.* Toronto, Canada: York University.

Daley, A. E., & MacDonnell, J. A. (2010, November). *Draft access and equity framework: Home care.* Paper presented to "Out" in Home Care Invitational Stakeholder workshop, Toronto, ON.

Daley, A. E., & MacDonnell, J. A. (2011). Gender, sexuality and the discursive representation of access and equity in health services literature: Implications for LGBT communities. *International Journal for Equity in Health, 10*(40), 1–10.

de Vries, B., & Croghan, C. F. (2014). LGBT aging: The contributions of community-based research. *Journal of Homosexuality, 61*(1), 1–20.

Erdley, S. D., Anklam, D. D., & Reardon, C. C. (2014). Breaking barriers and building bridges: Understanding the pervasive needs of older LGBT adults and the value of social work in health care. *Journal of Gerontological Social Work, 57*(2–4), 362–385.

Fabbre, V. D. (2014). Gender transitions in later life: The significance of time in queer aging. *Journal of Gerontological Social Work, 57*(2–4), 161–175.

Finkenauer, S., Sherratt, J., Marlow, J., & Brodey, A. (2012). When injustice gets old: A systematic review of trans aging. *Journal of Gay and Lesbian Social Services, 24*(4), 311–330.

Fredriksen-Goldsen, K. I., Hoy-Ellis, C. P., Goldsen, J., Emlet, C. A., & Hooyman, N. R. (2014). Creating a vision for the future: Key competencies and strategies for culturally competent practice with lesbian, gay, bisexual, and transgender (LGBT) older adults in the health and human services. *Journal of Gerontological Social Work, 57*(2–4), 80–107.

Fredriksen-Goldsen, K. I., Hyun-Jun, K., Barkan, S. E., Muraco, A., & Hoy-Ellis, C. P. (2013). Health disparities among lesbian, gay, and bisexual older adults: Results from a population-based study. *American Journal of Public Health, 103*(10), 1802–1809.

Gardner, A. T., de Vries, B., & Mockus, D. S. (2014). Aging out in the desert: Disclosure, acceptance, and service use among midlife and older lesbians and gay men. *Journal of Homosexuality*, *61*(1), 129–144.

Geary, C. R., & Schumacher, K. L. (2012). Care transitions: Integrating transition theory and complexity science concepts. *Advances in Nursing Science, 35*(3), 236–248.

Graham, C. L, Ivey, S. L., & Neuhauser, L. (2009). From hospital to home: Assessing the transitional care needs of vulnerable seniors. *The Gerontologist, 49*(1), 23–33.

Gratwick, S., Jihanian, L. J., Holloway, I. W., Sanchez, M., & Sullivan, K. (2014). Social work practice with LGBT seniors. *Journal of Gerontological Social Work, 57*(8), 889–907.

Gabrielson, M. L. (2011a). "We have to create family": Aging support issues and needs among older lesbians. *Journal of Gay and Lesbian Social Services, 23*(3), 322–334.

Gabrielson, M. L. (2011b). "I will not be discriminated against": Older lesbians creating new communities. *Advances in Nursing Science, 34*(4), 357–373.

Grigorovich, A. (2015a). The meaning of quality of care in home care settings: Older lesbian and bisexual women's perspectives. *Scandinavian Journal of Caring Sciences.* http://dx.doi.org/10.1111/scs.12228

Grigorovich, A. (2015b). Negotiating sexuality in home care settings: Older lesbians and bisexual women's experiences. *Culture, Health & Sexuality: An International Journal for Research, Intervention and Care, 17*(8), 947–961.

Grigorovich, A. (2015c). Restricted access: Older lesbian and bisexual women's experiences with home care services. *Research on Aging, 37*(7), 763–783.

Grollman, E. A. (2012, January 12). *What is transphobia? And what is cissexism.* Kinsey Sexual Health Information, Kinsey Institute. Retrieved from http://kinseyconfidential.org/transphobia

Gutman, G., & Spencer, C. (Eds.). (2010). *Aging, ageism and abuse: Moving from awareness to action*. Amsterdam: Elsevier.

Hardacker, C. T., Rubinstein, B., Hotton, A., & Houlberg, M. (2014). Adding silver to the rainbow: The development of the nurses' health education about LGBT elders (HEALE) cultural competency curriculum. *Journal of Nursing Management, 22*(2), 257–266.

Harley, D. A., & Teaster, P. B. (Eds.). (2016). *Handbook of LGBT elders: An interdisciplinary approach to principles, practices, and policies*. New York, NY: Springer Publishing.

Hovey, J. E. (2009). Nursing wounds: Why LGBT elders need protection from discrimination and abuse based on sexual orientation and gender identity. *Elder Law Journal, 17*, 93–106.

Hughes, A. K., Harold, R. D., & Boyer, J. M. (2011). Awareness of LGBT aging issues among aging services network providers. *Journal of Gerontological Social Work, 54*(7), 659–677.

Impact Report: LGBT Age Capacity Building Project. (2015, June). Retrieved from http://www.lgbthealth.org.uk/wp-content/uploads/2015/01/Impact-Report.pdf

Institute of Medicine. (2011). *The health of lesbian, gay, bisexual, and transgender people: Building a foundation for better understanding*. Washington, DC: The National Academies Press.

Kimmel, D. (2014). Lesbian, gay, bisexual, and transgender ageing concerns. *Clinical Gerontologist, 37*(1), 49–63.

Knauer, N. J. (2011). 'Gen Silent': Advocating for LGBT Elders. *Elder Law Journal, 19*, 101.

Knochel, K. A., Croghan, C. F., Moone, R. P., & Quam, J. K. (2012). Training, geography, and provision of aging services to lesbian, gay, bisexual, and transgender older adults. *Journal of Gerontological Social Work, 55*(5), 426–443.

Lee, E. O. J., & Brotman, S. (2011). Identity, refugeeness, belonging: Experiences of sexual minority refugees in Canada. *Canadian Review of Sociology, 48*(3), 241–274.

Leyva, V. L., Breshears, E. M., & Ringstad, R. (2014). Assessing the efficacy of LGBT cultural competency training for aging services providers in California's Central Valley. *Journal of Gerontological Social Work, 57*(2–4), 335–348.

LGBT-Age-Audit-Tool (2015): *A guide for services and organizations working with older people to become more LGBT inclusive*. Retrieved from http://www.lgbthealth.org.uk/wp-content/uploads/2015/09/LGBT-Age-Audit-Tool-final.pdf

Lim, F. A., & Bernstein, I. (2012). Promoting awareness of LGBT issues in aging in a baccalaureate nursing program. *Nursing Education Perspectives, 33*(3), 170–175.

MacDonnell, J. A., & Daley, A. (2015). Examining the development of positive space in health and social service organizations: A Canadian exploratory study. *Journal of Gay and Lesbian Social Services, 27*(3), 263–301.

Maddux, S. (Producer & Director). (2011). *Gen silent–The LGBT aging film* [Documentary]. United States: Interrobang! Productions.

McCann, E., Sharek, D., Higgins, A., Sheerin, F., & Glacken, M. (2013). Lesbian, gay, bisexual and transgender older people in Ireland: Mental health issues. *Aging and Mental Health, 17*(3), 358–365.

McCourt, P. (2008). *Promoting seniors' wellbeing: The seniors' mental health policy lens toolkit.* Victoria, BC: BC Psychogeriatric Association.

McGill, N. (2014). Advocates raise awareness of range of LGBT health issues: Programs address disparities, needs. *The Nation's Health, 44*(5), 1–14.

McGovern, J. (2014). The forgotten: Dementia and the aging LGBT community. *Journal of Gerontological Social Work, 57*(8), 845–857.

Meyer, H. (2011). Federal policy, activism, and LGBT older adults. *Temple Political and Civil Rights Law Review, 21*, 511.

Moore, D. (2009). Designing long-term care for lesbian, gay, bisexual, transsexual and transgender people. In P. Armstrong, M. Boscoe, B. Claw, K. Grant, M. Haworth-Brockman, B. Jackson, et al. (Eds.), *A place to call home: Long-term care in Canada* (pp. 104–110). Halifax, Canada: Fernwood Publishing.

Morales, M. J., King, M. D., Hiler, H., Coopwood, M. S., & Wayland, S. (2014). The greater St. Louis LGBT health and human services needs assessment: An examination of silent and baby boom generations. *Journal of Homosexuality, 61*(1), 103–128.

Muraco, A., & Fredriksen-Goldsen, K. (2011). "That's what friends do": Informal caregiving for chronically ill lesbian, gay, and bisexual elders. *Journal of Social and Personal Relationships, 28*(8), 1073–1092.

Murray, E., Numer, M., Merritt, B. Gahagan, J., & Comber, S. (2011). Healthy aging among LGBT seniors in Canada: A review of the literature. *International Journal of Health, Wellness and Society, 1*(4).

National Gay and Lesbian Task Force. (2005). *Make room for all: Diversity, cultural competency and discrimination in an aging America.* Retrieved from http://www.thetaskforce.org/static_html/downloads/reports/reports/MakeRoomForAll.pdf

Neville, S., & Henrickson, M. (2010). 'Lavender retirement': A questionnaire survey of lesbian, gay, and bisexual people's accommodation plans for old age. *International Journal of Nursing Practice, 16*(6), 586–594.

Ontario Home Care Association. (2014). *Facts and figures: Publically funded home care.* Retrieved from http://www.homecareontario.ca/home-care-services/facts-figures/publiclyfundedhomecare

Orel, N. A. (2014). Investigating the needs and concerns of lesbian, gay, bisexual, and transgender older adults: The use of qualitative and quantitative methodology. *Journal of Homosexuality, 61*(1), 53–78.

Peate, I. (2015). Caring for older lesbian, gay and bisexual people. *British Journal of Community Nursing, 18*(8), 372–374.

Porter, K. E., & Krinsky, L. (2014). Do LGBT aging trainings effectuate positive change in mainstream elder service providers? *Journal of Homosexuality, 61*(1), 197–216.

Portz, J. D., Retrum, J. H., Wrights, L. A., Boggs, J. M., Wilkins, S., Grimm, C., et al. (2014). Assessing capacity for providing culturally competent services to LGBT older adults. *Journal of Gerontological Social Work, 57*(2–4), 305–321.

Rawlings, D. (2012). End-of-life care considerations for gay, lesbian, bisexual, and transgender individuals. *International Journal of Palliative Nursing, 18*(1), 29–34.

Registered Nurses Association of Ontario. (2007). *Respecting sexual orientation and gender identity* [Position statement]. Toronto, ON.

River, L. (2006). *A feasibility study of the needs of older lesbians in Camden and surrounding boroughs.* Retrieved from http://www.ageofdiversity.org.uk/sites/default/files/OlderLesbianReport.pdf

Rosenfeld, D. (2003). *The Changing of the guard: Lesbian and gay elders, identity, and social change.* Philadelphia, PA: Temple University Press.

Rowan, N. L., & Giunta, N. (2014). Building capacity in gerontological social work for lesbian, gay, bisexual, and transgender older adults and their loved ones. *Journal of Gerontological Social Work, 57*(2–4), 75–79.

Schwinn, S. V., & Dinkel, S. A. (2015). Changing the culture of long-term care: Combating heterosexism. *Online Journal of Issues in Nursing, 20*(2).

Sears, J. T. (Ed.). (2013). *Growing older: Perspectives on LGBT aging.* New York, NY: Routledge.

Simone, M. J., & Appelbaum, J. S. (2011). Addressing the needs of older lesbian, gay, bisexual, and transgender adults. *Clinical Geriatrics, 19*(2), 38–45.

Sinding, C. (1999). Counting on desire: Supporting a lesbian with breast cancer. In M. Denton, M. Hadjukowski-Ahmed, M. O'Connor, & I. U. Zeytinoglu (Eds.), *Women's voices in health promotion* (pp. 191–203). Toronto, ON: Canadian Scholar's Press.

Siverskog, A. (2014). "They just don't have a clue": Transgender aging and implications for social work. *Journal of Gerontological Social Work, 57*(2–4), 386–406.

Stein, G. L., Beckerman, N. L., & Sherman, P. A. (2010). Lesbian and gay elders and long-term care: Identifying the unique psychosocial perspectives and challenges. *Journal of Gerontological Social Work, 53*(5), 412–435.

Stonewall. (2011). *Lesbian, gay and bisexual people in later life.* Retrieved from http://www.stonewall.org.uk/documents/lgb_in_later_life_final.pdf

Sullivan, K. M. (2014). Acceptance in the domestic environment: The experience of senior housing for lesbian, gay, bisexual, and transgender seniors. *Journal of Gerontological Social Work, 57*(2–4), 235–250.

Swan, W. (2014). Data-driven health care and senior care analysis. In W. Swan (Ed.), *Gay, lesbian, bisexual, and transgender civil rights: A public policy agenda for uniting a divided America* (pp. 191–198). Boca Raton, FL: CRC Press.

Tinney, J., Dow, B., Maude, P., Purchase, R., Whyte, C., & Barrett, C. (2015). Mental health issues and discrimination among older LGBTI people. *International Psychogeriatrics, 27*(9), 1411–1416.

Turcotte, M., & Schellenberg, G. (2007). *A Portrait of Seniors in Canada: 2006.* Ottawa: Statistics Canada. Retrieved from http://publications.gc.ca/Collection/Statcan/89-519-X/89-519-XIE2006001.pdf

Van Sluytman, L. G., & Torres, D. (2014). Hidden or uninvited? A content analysis of elder LGBT of color literature in gerontology. *Journal of Gerontological Social Work, 57*(2–4), 130–160.

Van Wagenen, A., Driskell, J., & Bradford, J. (2013). "I'm still raring to go": Successful aging among lesbian, gay, bisexual, and transgender older adults. *Journal of Aging Studies, 27*(1), 1–14.

Vermette, L., & Godin, G. (1996). Nurses' intentions to provide home care: The impact of AIDS and homosexuality. *AIDS Care*, *8*(4), 479–488.

Ward, R., River, L., & Fenge, L.-A. (2008). Neither silent nor invisible: A comparison of two participative projects involving older lesbians and gay men in the United Kingdom. *Journal of Gay and Lesbian Social Services, 20*(1–2), 147–165.

Westwood, S., King, A., Almack, K., Suen, Y. T., & Bailey, L. (2015). Good practice in health and social care provision for older LGBT people in the UK. In J. Fish & K. Karban (Eds.), *Lesbian, gay, bisexual and trans health inequalities: International perspectives in social work* (pp. 145–158). Chicago, IL: Policy Press.

Witten, T. M., & Eyler, A. E. (2012). Transgender and aging: Beings and becomings. In T. M. Witten & A. E. Eyler (Eds.), *Gay, lesbian, bisexual and transgender aging: Challenges in research, practice and policy* (pp. 187–269). New York, NY: The John Hopkins University Press.

Woody, I. (2014). Aging out: A qualitative exploration of ageism and heterosexism among aging African American lesbians and gay men. *Journal of Homosexuality, 61*(1), 145–165.

Wright, L., Grimm, C., Retrum, J. H., Helander, K., Wilkins, S., Boggs, J., et al. (2014). B3-4: Establishing an aging-in-place model for the lesbian, gay, bisexual, and transgender (LGBT) community: Lessons learned from a community-research partnership. *Clinical Medicine and Research*, *12*(1–2), 106.

Zodikoff, B. (2006). Services for lesbian, gay, bisexual and transgender older adults. In B. Berkman & S. D'Ambruoso (Eds.), *Handbook of social work in health and aging* (pp. 569–576). New York, NY: Oxford University Press.

CHAPTER 11

The Impact of Public Policy on LGBT Aging

Kenneth T. South

ABSTRACT

Until recently, there has been little recognition of the unique needs of lesbian, gay, bisexual, and transgender (LGBT) elders and even fewer accommodations provided for them through federal, state, and local public policy initiatives. This chapter provides an overview of the most recent policy successes for the LGBT community in general and for LGBT elders in particular. The LGBT elder population is currently the largest ever seen and its numbers will continue to grow as the "boomer" generation affects the entire U.S. population. It also describes the public policy work that has yet to be done by concerned advocates, activists, and allies. Readers will come away with a new appreciation of the diversity within the LGBT elder population as well as a deeper understanding of the historic and current struggles they face in seeking a fulfilling life, in spite of a history of prejudice and injustice.

INTRODUCTION

> "Morality cannot be legislated, but behavior can be regulated. Judicial decrees may not change the heart, but they can restrain the heartless."
>
> —Martin Luther King, Jr.

http://dx.doi.org/10.1891/0198-8794.37.161

Until recently, there has been little recognition of the unique needs of lesbian, gay, bisexual, and transgender (LGBT) elders and even fewer accommodations provided for them through federal, state, and local public policy initiatives. With the impact of their exponential growth in numbers and the visibility and impact of the baby boomer generation, change has been, and is being, accomplished. While the positive, creative, and thoughtful legislative actions that have included LGBT elders are to be commended, there remains the reality of the destructive nature of homophobia, transphobia, sexism, racism, and ageism, which impacts every aspect of the daily lives of LGBT people of all ages. This chapter describes the public policy efforts that have been achieved to incorporate LGBT elders as full members of society, including policies around same-sex marriage and the Affordable Care Act (ACA), as well as future policy directions for this population.

BACKGROUND

The baby boomer generation in America (born between 1946 and 1964; Freedman, 1999) has already had an enormous impact on all levels of society. The current population of LGBT elders is also larger now than it ever has been. Public policy, however, has not always recognized this group as a special population or recognized their unique needs. While LGBT elders enjoy some of the same benefits as their fellow seniors because of their age, there are significant differences between these populations that demand particular attention.

LGBT seniors now approaching their retirement years are the first generation to live most of their lives openly within a society that spent hundreds of years defining them as criminals, pedophiles, mentally ill, or those who chose to live a deviant lifestyle and not conform to the standards of mainstream society. LGBT elders continue to live in a society that tells them they are "different," and are "outsiders" and survive among homophobia and prejudice that ranges from total ignorance to violence and even homicide. Many have experienced rejection by family of origin and have felt the need to hide their true selves from family and friends. They also face legislated discrimination, as the United States still does not have an employment nondiscrimination law that includes gender identity or sexual orientation. LGBT elders also fear being the target of violence. In fact, a recent FBI Hate Crimes Statistics report issued in 2014 documents that the second largest number of violent crimes reported, 20.8%, were those committed on persons because of their sexual orientation (Federal Bureau of Investigation, 2014). Not surprisingly, this daily stress has been shown to cause serious effects on LGBT health in general, and LGBT elders' health in particular (Fredriksen-Goldsen et al., 2013; McCabe et al., 2010; Krieger, 2000).

In the past decade, progress has been made in recognizing the unique needs of this population and combating the discrimination that they face. One of the first of these efforts was the publication, *Outing Age, Public Policy Issues Affecting LGBT Elders* by the National Gay and Lesbian Taskforce (Cahill, South, & Spade, 2000). This groundbreaking publication analyzed the current state of affairs for older LGBT adults and called for 70 specific national and local policy changes to support LGBT elders. Since 2000, several of the "*Outing Age*" recommendations have become policy or law. Progress since 2000 has included the passage of the *Hate Crimes Prevention Act* in 2009; the *Ensuring Hospital Visitation Rights for LGBT Patients* by a presidential executive memo in 2010; and the enactment of the ACA. Also in 2010, the U.S. Department of Health and Human Services (DHHS) awarded a grant to Services and Advocacy for GLBT Elders (SAGE) to establish a National Resource Center on LGBT Aging. An amendment to prohibit LGBT discrimination in the Fair Housing Act was passed in 2012, and the *Defense of Marriage Act* (DOMA) was declared unconstitutional by the Supreme Court in 2013. In 2014, Presidential Executive Order #11246 was issued ensuring nondiscrimination of LGBT federal government employees, which included gender identity. Same-sex marriage was upheld by the Supreme Court in 2015, which fulfills numerous *Outing Age* recommendations. The *Older Americans Act* (OAA) was reauthorized in 2016, although the provisions called for by LGBT advocates were not included.

CURRENT POLICIES IMPACTING OLDER LGBTS

Same-Sex Marriage

On June 25, 2015, the U.S. Supreme Court announced its landmark decision in *Obergefell v. Hodges,* which guarantees same-sex couples the freedom to marry in all 50 states and requires all states to recognize same-sex marriages performed in other states. Despite this right, only a small percentage (approximately 9%) of the total LGBT population in the United States has chosen to marry (Gates, 2014, 2015). The total number of married LGBT elders is not known, but assumed to be a much smaller segment of this LGBT married population. This ruling has been the most impactful of recent policies pertaining to LGBTs. Earlier policies enacted by the Supreme Court, the Internal Revenue Service (IRS), and the DHHS also paved the way for more inclusive benefits and equal rights for same-sex couples.

On June 26, 2013, the U.S. Supreme Court struck down the section of the DOMA that previously barred same-sex couples from qualifying for each other's federal benefits. These benefits include Social Security survivor benefits, federal tax benefits, and employee health and retirement benefits. In light of the subsequent same-sex marriage decision, a spouse can now receive up to half of a living spouse's benefit, if it is larger than his or her own, and widows or widowers are now able to receive up to 100% of a deceased spouse's benefit or the choice of continuing his or her own benefit (Van Sluytman, 2013).

The Centers for Medicare & Medicaid Services, a division of the DHHS, issued an official Federal Policy Guidance on July 1, 2013, making it clear that same-sex partners must be given equal visitation rights at long-term care facilities, regardless of their marital status. This applies to all long-term care facilities receiving Medicare and Medicaid funding, including nursing homes and hospice facilities. All patients in these facilities must be given the right to receive visitors of their choosing, regardless of whether the patient and visitors have a legally recognized or biological relationship. It also explicitly states that discrimination against the same-sex spouse or partner seeking to visit a patient is prohibited (Rupert, 2013).

The IRS ruled on September 23, 2013 by *Notice 2013-61* (2013), same-sex couples, legally married in jurisdictions that recognized their marriages (which now include all married LGBT couples), will be treated as married for federal tax purposes. Therefore, same-sex married couples now have the same choice as the rest of the population to file jointly or separately as married. These couples now have multiple options to seek marriage benefits or in some cases, realize marriage penalties when they file their annual tax return.

Even though the issue of marriage may not affect the majority, it has raised the level of visibility for all LGBT elders and subsequently made major impacts on other areas of policy and entitlements such as Social Security, Medicare, and Medicaid. For example, Medicare enrollment requests for Special Enrollment Periods are administered by Social Security Administration (SSA, n.d.). Many of the requests for reductions in late-enrollment penalties are made by same-sex spouses. Eligibility for Medicare Part A, which covers hospitalizations, and Part B, which covers doctor visits, is particularly important for LGBT couples who are disproportionately likely to be uninsured. Part A coverage is often available without paying a monthly premium, making it all the more important for the many lesbian, gay, and bisexual elders for whom it can be challenging to afford these payments (Cray, 2014). Additionally, the Medicaid program has had a long-standing provision called "spousal protections." Many older Americans rely on Medicaid to pay the extremely high costs of long-term medical care. To be eligible for the Medicaid program, seniors must demonstrate that their financial assets are not over $2,000.00. The spousal protection provision in Medicaid does not count the couples' home as an asset, thus ensuring that the noninstitutional spouse will continue to have a place to live. Until the passage of the same-sex marriage law, this benefit was only available to heterosexual couples (Elder Law Answers, n.d.).

The Affordable Care Act

The ACA was passed by Congress and signed into law by President Obama on March 23, 2010 and on June 25, 2015 the Supreme Court case (*King v. Burwell*) rendered a final decision to uphold the constitutionality of the ACA (Hanel, 2015). The ACA is the most sweeping reform of the health care system in the United States since the introduction of Medicare and Medicaid under the "Great Society" legislation in the 1960s under President Lyndon Johnson (Helsing, 2000). It provides much needed benefits for all uninsured LGBT Americans and has particular benefits for LGBT elders. One specific provision of the program that eliminates the denial of insurance for people with "preexisting conditions" is particularly important to those with HIV or other chronic diseases. The law not only impacts individuals as they approach 65 when they can enroll in Medicare, but the ACA also provides for current Medicare recipients as well.

Other changes facilitated by the ACA benefit older adults of all sexual orientations and gender identities. One is the benefit of increased savings for medications for those whose annual costs fit into what has been called the "donut hole" in Medicare Part D—that is, out of pocket drug costs between $2,500 and $4,500 per year. While this "donut hole" will be entirely eliminated by 2020, thanks to the ACA, seniors can now receive a 50% discount on their medications, and Medicare now provides free annual wellness doctor visits as well as free coverage of important preventive services (Tax, 2015). Some elders are known as "dual eligible," receiving benefits from both Medicare and Medicaid. While most long-term care in nursing homes and similar institutions is paid for by Medicaid, new provisions in the ACA will now make it possible for some seniors to get increased benefits for home care services and therefore postpone their much more expensive long-term care arrangements. And because of the *Ensuring Hospital Visitation Rights for LGBT Patients* presidential executive memo of 2010, LGBT families and friends need no longer fear their rejection by institutional staff to visit their loved ones.

Family and Medical Leave Act

The Family and Medical Leave Act was an important accomplishment of the Clinton administration, signed into law by the president on February 5, 1993. It was a boon to millions of working Americans who had ill family members at home needing their attention and care. Like most legislation of its time, family and "spouses" were defined as blood relatives or legally married, heterosexual couples. With the Supreme Court decision on same-sex marriage, the U.S. Department of Labor on February 25, 2015 recognized same-sex couples on a par with their heterosexual married counterparts. Like them, LGBT spouses are now allowed up to 12 paid weeks of leave or 26 weeks of unpaid leave to care for a loved one (Moller, 2015).

The Matthew Shepard and James Byrd, Jr. Hate Crimes Prevention Act

This most recent revision of the 1969 Hate Crime Act was signed into law by President Obama on October 28, 2009. A hate crime is now defined as a violent act perpetrated against a person because of the real or perceived, religion, national origin, gender, *sexual orientation, gender identity*, or disability of that person. This protection is critical for LGBT people of all ages to stem the violence that has been all too common for LGBT people over the years, perpetrated because of the perceived or actual sexual orientation or gender identity of individuals (Leadership Conference, n.d.).

The Elder Justice Act

The National Center on Elder Abuse (NCEA), a division of the Office on Aging of the DHHS, outlines the common definition of the harmful acts perpetrated on one of the most vulnerable of groups in our society, older adults:

> In general, elder abuse refers to intentional or neglectful acts by a caregiver or "trusted" individual that lead to, or may lead to, harm of a vulnerable elder. Physical abuse; neglect; emotional or psychological abuse; verbal abuse and threats; financial abuse and exploitation; sexual abuse; and abandonment are considered forms of elder abuse. In many states, self-neglect is also considered mistreatment. (NCEA, n.d.)

The NCEA estimates that upwards of 10% of all elders 65+ have experienced some sort of this mistreatment in their lives (Teaster et al., 2004). When the elder in question is a lesbian, gay man, or transgendered person, the levels of abuse and maltreatment often increase dramatically. The NCEA and SAGE report that this percentage skyrockets to 65% for older LGBT adults, with upwards of 29% being physically attacked by caregivers. Older LGBT adults often endure this level of abuse primarily because of discrimination and bigotry, fueled by homophobia, transphobia, and sexism. Many LGBT elders over 65 lived during a time when and in contexts where disclosure of one's sexual orientation would have dire consequences, so "passing" as a heterosexual person meant survival from ridicule, loss of employment, institutionalization, incarceration, physical violence, and even death (Butler, 2004). And, research indicates that the number one fear of being admitted to a long-term care facility is the anxiety around being "found out" and the fear of being mistreated because of their sexual orientation (Hovey, 2009).

Social prejudice against transgendered persons is known as *transphobia*. It is a powerful force in the society that keeps trans people from living dignified lives in every way. Research points to high levels of victimization and violence toward transgendered people of all ages (National Center for Transgender Equality, 2014a).

Major barriers exist in obtaining a fair picture of trans elder abuse. Rather than reporting incidents of abuse and violence to the law enforcement and health care professionals, trans people have experienced routine levels of prejudice and violence at the hands of law enforcement and health care professionals (Cook-Daniels, 1998).

Because of the passage of the ACA, relief for LGBT elders may be found in its provisions within the Patient Protection section, which establishes the Elder Justice Act (Section 6702), signed into law by President Obama on March 23, 2010. It provides federal resources to "prevent, detect, treat, understand, intervene in and, where appropriate, prosecute elder abuse, neglect and exploitation" (Dong & Simon, 2011, p. 2461).

With its full implementation, the new law will help abused elders and prevent abuse by establishing two new national councils on elder abuse, supporting improvements in ombudsman programs, and increasing support for State Adult Protective Services programs. It also has an intensive focus on criminal abuse in long-term care facilities.

SPECIAL POLICY ISSUES FOR TRANSGENDER ELDERS

An Understanding of the Transgender Population Begins With Terminology

Transsexual refers to a person whose biological sex does not conform to their own understanding of their gender (Carroll, Gilroy, & Ryan, 2002). Many, if they can afford it, choose to have a sex reassignment surgery to create male or female genitalia, or enhance other parts of their body, to conform to their understanding of their gender. *Cross-dressers, formerly* "transvestites," refer to people who choose to wear the clothing of the opposite sex. These persons are not looking to change their given male or female sex. Some people cross-dress on an occasional, recreational basis; others may live their entire lives in this way (Blanchard, Racansky, & Steiner, 1986). *Intersexed* persons, formerly referred to as *hermaphrodites*, are people born with some combination of both male and female genitalia. Controversy continues to exist in the medical community about standards of care for this population. Some parents and doctors make a decision at birth as to which gender will be assigned to the child, while other health care professionals urge parents to wait for the child to reach adolescence before any intervention (Cohen-Kettenis, 2003; Diamond, 1997). *Gender-queer* is a term that refers to individuals or groups who "queer" or problematize the hegemonic notions of sex, gender, and desire in a given society" (University of Michigan, n.d.). Transgender has become widely used as a generic term for the whole community, also referred to as the "trans community" or "trans people." But it also refers to those people who do not find themselves in any single category, blending sex, sexual orientation, and gender. Recently, another term has come into use, which is "gender-nonconforming" people (Tillery, 2010).

When examining public policies related to LGBT older adults, it is critical to point out the lack of public policy protections for transgender elders. Additionally, there must be recognition that the general level of knowledge and understanding of this community is minimal. Not only are most American citizens ignorant of the realities of the daily lives of this diverse group, but even professionals responsible for providing health care and other services are often not fully sensitive to or informed of their special issues and needs. As a result, trans elders have faced numerous levels of discrimination and maltreatment over the course of their lives. Various studies over the years have looked at the treatment of trans elders in health care institutions, and all have found similar injustices at varying degrees of severity (Ritter, 2010; Eliason, 2010; Jackson, Johnson, & Roberts, 2008; Williams & Freeman 2007). For example, trans elders have been refused medical care, and many have found they have had to be the educators to their caregivers about trans issues (Stein, Beckerman, & Sherman, 2010).

Recent policy changes have advanced the rights of transgender elders to a small degree. In 2013, the SSA changed the policy for changing one's gender. In this change, the SSA has modernized the medical requirements required of trans people to update or change their gender in their social security records. The office also issued guidelines to all SSA employees, educating them on important protections such as confidentiality, proper pronoun usage, and how trans people should be engaged with respect and dignity (Lentini, 2013). Further, on September 3, 2015, the DHHS proposed new rules to add a nondiscrimination provision in the ACA, under Section 1557. The ruling made it illegal for participating insurance companies to refuse transsexuals who have chosen to have sex-reassignment surgery. However, this provision did not go far enough. A year before, on January 23, 2014, a consortium of organizations including: The Community of LGBT Centers, the Human Rights Campaign, FORGE (an organization serving trans survivors), Lambda Legal, National Center for Transgender Equality, the National Gay and Lesbian Task Force, and SAGE issued a statement that expressed outrage that DHHS had refused to include explicit nondiscrimination protections for LGBT and other consumers to Medicaid's Home and Community-Based Services program. It is this program that pays specifically for home care services, where mistreatment and discrimination of this population have been well-documented (National Center for Transgender Equality, 2014b).

FUTURE DIRECTIONS AND NEEDED CHANGES TO PUBLIC POLICY

The OAA, first established in 1965 as part of the "Great Society" initiatives of the Johnson Administration, is the primary program to serve millions of America's older adults with its two billion dollar annual authorization. It supports a range of home and community-based services, such as Meals on Wheels and other nutrition programs, in-home services, transportation, legal services, elder abuse prevention, and caregiver support. However, as mentioned previously, LGBT seniors have never been included in its legislative language (Baker & Krehely, 2011). For many years LGBT advocates have called for amendments to the law to target the unique needs of LGBT elders. The current version of the OAA became law number 114–144 when President Obama signed the legislation on April 19, 2016 (Congress.gov, n.d.). And again, unfortunately, the hard work of numerous advocates for LGBT older adults were again extremely disappointed when none of their recommended provisions were enacted. However, public policy progress does not depend on one piece of legislation during one administration; it must be seen in the long view. The need continues and the provisions previously recommended continue to provide valid goals for the future. Some of those provisions include:

- Designation of LGBT older adults as a vulnerable population with greatest economic and social need as a result of a lifetime of discrimination
- Permanent establishment of the National Resource Center on LGBT Aging, the country's first and only technical assistance resource center aimed at improving the quality of services and supports offered to LGBT older adults
- Improvement of data collection and analysis on the effectiveness of the state units on aging and the Area Agencies on Aging in targeting services to LGBT older adults
- Prioritization of research and development grants for organizations working to improve LGBT health, long-term care needs, and access to culturally responsive services (National Council on Aging, n.d.).

As previously mentioned, *Outing Age 2010: Public Policy Issues Affecting Gay, Lesbian, Bisexual, and Transgender Elders* (Grant, Koskovich, Frazer, & Bjerk, 2010) was published as an updated revision of the same publication released in 2000. While some of the 21 key recommendations have since been accomplished, there are several major tasks for advocates to address. Among them are:

- Amend the OAA to require funded agencies to collect research data on LGBT elders.
- Pass The *Equality Act* (S. 1858 introduced on July 23, 2015), which establishes explicit, permanent protections against discrimination based on an individual's sexual orientation or gender identity in matters of employment, housing, access to public places, federal funding, credit, education, and jury service (Ford, 2015).
- Fund programs that will specifically target the social isolation of LGBT elders by supporting LGBT-specific friendly visitor programs.

HOW TO AFFECT POLICY CHANGE

Professionals in the health care field are not only responsible for providing the best care possible to their clients, but they are also important players in the public policy advocacy arena. However, since many in this field are employed by nonprofit organizations they may be concerned that if they engage in "lobbying" for a cause they believe in, they could jeopardize the nonprofit status of the organization. This is very seldom the case. The definition of "lobbying" used by the IRS is very specific and rather narrow; few professionals who are interested in advocating for better public policy for their clients would meet this definition (Duke Medicine, n.d.).

Most new legislation or public policy change happens in the United States because of the efforts of many individuals. An example would be the women's suffrage movement, an effort that started with the pioneering work of Susan B. Anthony in 1837 and resulted in the passage of the Nineteenth Amendment to the Constitution, which finally gave women the right to vote after a 74-year struggle (Heinemann, S. 1996). Not all new public policy efforts take 74 years to move from the recognition of a need to the creation of a law or governmental policy to respond to that need. But the process to get there is pretty much the same. To get there partnerships must be developed among activists, government relations offices, advocates, associations, as well as grass roots voters, and state or federal legislative offices and their public officials. And the process can start from any one of these partners. There are several steps professionals can take to get involved:

- Contact national or state professional association "government affairs" staff and inquire as to their involvement with LGBT policy issues.

- Inquire within home institutions as to their cultural sensitivity to LGBT elders' issues.
- Join a national organization that advocates for LGBT elders like SAGE, The Human Rights Campaign, The National Gay and Lesbian Taskforce, Lambda Legal, or the National Center for Transgender Equality.
- Support local LGBT advocacy organizations to be better informed of the cutting edge issues in the community.

Since 2000, there have been numerous public policy efforts that have not only increased the visibility of LGBT elders but that have improved their lives significantly. Organizations providing direct services to LGBT elders have increased as have mainstream senior organizations that increasingly recognize LGBT elders already in their midst. The federal government, especially the Obama Administration, has accomplished more for LGBT seniors than any other previous administration. And, mainstream media has found this "invisible" population by including them in their coverage. A glance into the future tells us that LGBT elders will approach 3 million by 2030 (SAGE, 2010). Efforts to address the gaps in public policy remain enormous. Perhaps the legislative and policy changes of the past will provide inspiration for the work to come.

REFERENCES

Baker, K., & Krehely, J. (2011). How health care reform will help LGBT elders. *Public Policy and Aging Report, 21*(3), 19–23. Retrieved from https://www.sageusa.org/files/baker_ppar.pdf

Blanchard, R., Racansky, I. G., & Steiner, B. W. (1986). Phallometric detection of fetishistic arousal in heterosexual male cross-dressers. *Journal of Sex Research, 22*(4), 452–462.

Butler, S. S. (2004). Gay, lesbian, bisexual, and transgender (GLBT) elders: The challenges and resilience of this marginalized group. *Journal of Human Behavior in the Social Environment, 9*(4), 25–44.

Cahill, S., South, K., & Spade, J. (2000). *Outing age: Public policy issues affecting gay, lesbian, bisexual and transgender elders*. Washington, DC: Policy Institute of the National Gay and Lesbian Task Force.

Carroll, L., Gilroy, P. J., & Ryan, J. (2002). Counseling transgendered, transsexual, and gender-variant clients. *Journal of Counseling and Development, 80*(2), 131–139.

Cohen-Kettenis, P. T., & Pfäfflin, F. (2003). *Transgenderism and intersexuality in childhood and adolescence: Making choices* (Vol. 46). Thousand Oaks, CA: SAGE.

Congress.gov. (n.d.). *S.192 - Older Americans Act of 2016*. Retrieved from https://www.congress.gov/bill/114th-congress/senate-bill/192/committees

Cook-Daniels, L. (1998). Lesbian, gay male, bisexual and transgendered elders: Elder abuse and neglect issues. *Journal of Elder Abuse and Neglect, 9*(2), 35–49.

Cray, A. (2014, April 3). *Same-sex spouses now recognized for Medicare eligibility and enrollment, Think Progress*. Retrieved from http://thinkprogress.org/lgbt/2014/04/03/3422602/medicare-same-sex-couples

Diamond, M., & Sigmundson, H. K. (1997). Management of intersexuality: Guidelines for dealing with persons with ambiguous genitalia. *Archives of Pediatrics and Adolescent Medicine, 151*(10), 1046–1050.

Dong, X., & Simon, M. A. (2011). Enhancing national policy and programs to address elder abuse. *The Journal of the American Medical Association, 305*(23), 2460–2461.

Duke Medicine. (n.d.). *Lobbying definitions, exceptions, and examples*. Retrieved from https://governmentrelations.duke.edu/wp-content/uploads/2013/05/DefinitionsExceptionsExamples-2-12.pdf

Elder Law Answers. (n.d.). *Medicaid protections*. Retrieved from http://www.elderlawanswers.com/medicaid-protections-for-the-healthy-spouse-12019

Eliason, M. J., Dibble, S., & DeJoseph, J. (2010). Nursing's silence on lesbian, gay, bisexual, and transgender issues: The need for emancipatory efforts. *Advances in Nursing Science, 33*(3), 206–218.

Federal Bureau of Investigation. (2014). *Latest hate crime statistics report released*. Retrieved from https://www.fbi.gov/news/stories/latest-hate-crime-statistics-report-released/latest-hate-crime-statistics-report-released

Ford, J. (2015, July 23). *The Equality Act could end legal LGBT discrimination for good*. Retrieved from http://thinkprogress.org/lgbt/2015/07/23/3683728/equality-act-introduction

Fredriksen-Goldsen, K. I., Emlet, C. A., Kim, H. J., Muraco, A., Erosheva, E. A., Goldsen, J., et al. (2013). The physical and mental health of lesbian, gay male, and bisexual (LGB) older adults: The role of key health indicators and risk and protective factors. *The Gerontologist, 53*(4), 664–675.

Freedman, M. (1999). *Prime time: How baby boomers will revolutionize retirement and transform America*. New York, NY: Public Affairs.

Gates, G. J. (2014). *LGBT Demographics: Comparisons among population-based surveys*. Los Angeles, CA: The Williams Institute, UCLA School of Law. Retrieved from http://williamsinstitute.law.ucla.edu/wp-content/uploads/lgbt-demogs-sep-2014.pdf

Gates, G. J., & Newport, F. (2015, April 24). *An estimated 780,000 Americans in same-sex marriages*. Retrieved from http://www.gallup.com/poll/182837/estimated-780-000-americans-sex-marriages.aspx

Grant, J. M., Koskovich, G., Frazer, S., & Bjerk, S. (2010). *Outing age 2010: Public policy issues affecting gay, lesbian, bisexual, and transgender elders*. National Gay and Lesbian Task Force. Retrieved from http://www.lgbtagingcenter.org/resources/resource.cfm?r=30

Hanel, J. (2015, June). *King v. Burwell*. Retrieved from http://www.coloradohealthinstitute.org/uploads/downloads/King_v_Burwell_Decision.pdf

Heinemann, S. (1996). *Timelines of American women's history*. New York, NY: Penguin Books.

Helsing, J. W. (2000). *Johnson's war/Johnson's great society: The guns and butter trap.* Santa Barbara, CA: Greenwood Publishing Group.

Hovey, J. E. (2009). Nursing wounds: Why LGBT elders need protection from discrimination and abuse based on sexual orientation and gender identity. *Elder Law Journal*, *17*, 95.

Internal Revenue Service. (2013, August 29). *IRS announces that all legal same-sex marriages will be recognized for federal tax purposes and 3B ruling provides certainty, benefits and protections under federal tax law for same-sex married couples.* Retrieved from https://www.irs.gov/uac/newsroom/treasury-and-irs-announce-that-all-legal-same-sex-marriages-will-be-recognized-for-federal-tax-purposes-ruling-provides-certainty-benefits-and-protections-under-federal-tax-law-for-same-sex-married-couples

Jackson, N. C., Johnson, M. J., & Roberts, R. (2008). The potential impact of discrimination fears of older gays, lesbians, bisexuals and transgender individuals living in small- to moderate-sized cities on long-term health care. *Journal of Homosexuality*, *54*(3), 325–339.

Krieger, N. (2000). Discrimination and health. *Social Epidemiology*, *1*, 36–75.

Leadership Conference. (n.d.). *The Matthew Shepard and James Byrd, Jr. Hate Crimes Prevention Act.* Leadership Conference on Civil and Human Rights. Retrieved from http://www.civilrights.org/hatecrimes/llehcpa

Lentini, K. (2013, June 14). *Huge win Social Security Administration modernizes gender marker policy.* NGLTF Policy Institute. Retrieved from http://www.thetaskforce.org/huge-win-social-security-administration-modernizes-gender-marker-policy/

McCabe, S. E., Bostwick, W. B., Hughes, T. L., West, B. T., & Boyd, C. J. (2010). The relationship between discrimination and substance use disorders among lesbian, gay, and bisexual adults in the United States. *American Journal of Public Health*, *100*(10), 1946–1952.

Moller, J. (2015, March 4). *LGBT rights finally come to the FMLA.* Law 360. Retrieved from http://www.law360.com/articles/627072/lgbt-rights-finally-come-to-the-fmla

National Center for Transgender Equality. (2014a, January 14). *Transgender terminology.* Retrieved from http://www.transequality.org/issues/resources/transgender-terminology

National Center for Transgender Equality. (2014b, January 23). *LGBT advocates disappointed rules for community care fail to protect LGBT seniors.* Retrieved from http://www.transequality.org/blog/lgbt-advocates-disappointed-rules-for-community-care-fail-to-protect-lgbt-seniors

National Center on Elder Abuse. (n.d.). *Why should I care about elder abuse?* Retrieved from http://www.ncea.aoa.gov/Resources/Publication/docs/NCEA_WhyCare_508.pdf

National Council on Aging. (n.d.). *S. 192, Older Americans Act Reauthorization Act of 2015.* Retrieved from http://www.ncoa.org/public-policy-action/older-americans-act/senate/s-192

Ritter, M. J. (2010). Quality care for queer nursing home residents: The prospect of reforming the Nursing Home Reform Act. *Tex. L. Rev.*, *89*, 999.

Rupert, M. (2013, July 1). *New guidance from HHS protects LGBT elders, National center for lesbian rights*. Retrieved from http://www.nclrights.org/press-room/press-release/new-guidance-from-hhs-protects-lgbt-elders

SAGE. (2010, April 1). *Improving the lives of LGBT older adults*. Retrieved from http://www.sageusa.org/resources/publications.cfm?ID=17#sthash.fYFR8oFI.dpuf

Social Security Administration. (n.d.). *Compilation of the Social Security laws*. Retrieved from https://www.ssa.gov/OP_Home/ssact/title18/1837.htm

Stein, G. L., Beckerman, N. L., & Sherman, P. A. (2010). Lesbian and gay elders and long-term care: Identifying the unique psychosocial perspectives and challenges. *Journal of Gerontological Social Work*, *53*(5), 421–435.

Tax, A. (2015). *The Older Americans Act*. SAGE (Senior Advocacy for GLBT Elders), USA. Retrieved from https://www.SAGE (Senior Advocacy for GLBT Elders) https://sage-usa.org/issues/oaa.cfm

Teaster, P. B., Dugar, T., Mendiondo, M., Abner E. L., Cecil, K. A., & Otto J. M. (2004). *The 2004 survey of adult protective services: Abuse of adults 60 years of age and older*. National Center on Elder Abuse. Retrieved from http://www.ncea.aoa.gov/Resources/Publication/docs/APS_2004NCEASurvey.pdf

Tillery, B. (2010). *When health care Isn't caring: Lambda Legal's survey of discrimination against LGBT people and people with HIV*. Lambda Legal. Retrieved from http://www.lambdalegal.org/publications/when-health-care-isnt-caring

University of Michigan. (n.d.). *LGBT terms and definitions*. Retrieved from https://internationalspectrum.umich.edu/life/definitions

Van Sluytman, Laurens, G. (August 2013). *Shining a light on Medicare: Demystifying Medicare for the elder LGBT community*. Retrieved from https://www.lgbtagingcenter.org/resources/print.cfm?r=600

Williams, M. E., & Freeman, P. A. (2007). Transgender health: Implications for aging and caregiving. *Journal of Gay and Lesbian Social Services*, *18*(3–4), 93–108.

CHAPTER 12

Conclusion and Future Directions

Anissa Rogers and Kristina M. Hash

ABSTRACT

This chapter summarizes and concludes the volume. It reviews the literature on older LGBT adults, including what is known about the health, mental health, caregiving, and social supports of older LGBT adults. The chapter also includes a summary of best practices for work with this population as well as what is still needed by way of service, research, and policy considerations to increase the quality of services and reduce service barriers for older LGBT adults. Last, service, research, and policy recommendations are offered in an effort to improve service access and provision to older LGBT adults, with the ultimate goal of improving the health and well-being of those in this population.

INTRODUCTION

As the chapters in this volume reflect, society continues to progress in its attitudes toward LGBT persons, which has resulted in the development of many LGBT-friendly policies and services that strive to improve the lives of all LGBT individuals. Consequently, great strides have been made in improving the lives and well-being of older LGBT adults. Still, many challenges and barriers exist for these individuals, and there is much work to be done to better understand how to address these challenges and establish best practices for work in these communities. In particular, many gaps still exist in the literature with regard to the needs of older LGBT adults and the ways in which individuals navigate their

http://dx.doi.org/10.1891/0198-8794.37.175

diverse and complex situations and how service systems can best respond to the varied needs and harness the strengths of these individuals. In this concluding chapter, a summary of the research presented in the previous chapters is offered as well as suggestions for best practices for older LGBT adults and future directions for research and policy.

SUMMARY OF RESEARCH ON OLDER LGBT ADULTS

Physical, Mental, and Sexual Health of Older LGBT Adults

Many gaps in health care and health disparities exist for older LGBT adults. Among the many issues that persist, institutionalized discrimination and intersectional forms of oppression that disproportionately affect poor, minority older LGBT adults are still serious problems that create barriers to accessing health care and perpetuate health inequities. This is particularly true for individuals who are aging and face increased risk for disability and chronic illness and who often prefer to remain at home as they age. For older LGBT adults, health issues are often made worse by lifelong experiences with homophobic, biphobic, and transphobic stigma (Institute of Medicine, 2011).

A lack of education and training among health care professionals contribute to existing barriers and health care disparities for older LGBT adults. Older LGBT adults often avoid health care services because of experiences of violence, discrimination, and feelings of invisibility due to a lack of provider awareness of the unique issues faced by those in this population (e.g., Witten & Eyler, 2012). Advances that have been made in health care services for older LGBT adults often have not helped transgender adults or poor or ethnic minority LGBT adults who often face interlocking forms of oppression and multiple barriers to health care services (Chiplin, Chin, Dayton, Redman, & McIntyre, 2011).

Older LGBT adults also experience higher rates of mental distress than their non-LGBT counterparts. As with the health care environment, a long history of ageism, violence, stigmatization, and discriminatory behaviors and policies in mental health care settings has compromised the mental health of older LGBT adults, including access to mental health services (Hash & Rogers, 2013). Many older LGBT adults were subjected to lobotomies, castration, and reparative therapies, among other cruel interventions, because of their sexual identities, which were deemed mental illnesses (Fredriksen-Goldsen, Hoy-Ellis, Goldsen, Emlet, & Hooyman, 2014). Further, factors such as age, income, culture, minority stress, and internalized homophobia often contribute to mental health issues for older LGBT adults (King & Richardson, 2015).

Little is known about sexual health and satisfaction for older LGBT adults, particularly in relation to physical issues such as illness, medication use, or other risk factors associated with advancing age that may impede sexual health and contribute to sexual dysfunction. Even less is known about the sexual health and satisfaction of older transgender adults. The oldest-old LGBT adults are significantly less likely than their younger peers to disclose their sexual orientation or any history of discrimination (e.g., physical, psychological, or sexual abuse) to care providers and are less likely to receive appropriate sexual health assessment or treatment (Fredriksen-Goldsen, Kim, Shiu, Goldsen, & Emlet, 2015).

Factors contributing to a lack of knowledge about sexual health and dysfunction for older LGBT adults include institutionalized discrimination in health care systems, which often leads to a lack of outreach to minority populations as well as a lack of trust among older adults in health care providers. Further, a lack of attention to the diversity within the older LGBT population and a concomitant deficiency of rigor in research methods to study sexual health issues often lead to health disparities for those in subpopulations among the older LGBT community. For example, most surveys that do exist focus upon the sexual activity of gay and lesbian elders; no national surveys are available to provide detailed information about the sexual activity of older bisexual and transgender adults.

Bisexual and Transgender Older Adults

Older bisexual adults face biphobia, which can have profound effects on the health, mental health, and well-being of these individuals, and research on these issues is still scarce. Examining the intersectionality of factors such as race, class, and ethnicity with health and mental health outcomes is an important step in improving the well-being of older LGBT adults, particularly older bisexual and transgender adults who may face additional stigma and isolation (Bowleg, 2012).

Older bisexual adults may be shielded more from stereotypes than their younger counterparts, since their sexual orientation may be seen as more mature and less transitory; however, they may be more likely to internalize stereotypes and be invisible to others inside and outside of their communities. Further, older bisexual adults may face discrimination from others in the gay and lesbian community as well as from their families, service providers, and social communities. In addition, the concept of bisexuality is relatively new; thus, some older bisexual adults may not have had access to this term in their younger years and may be reluctant to adopt the term to define themselves (Scherrer, Kazyak, & Schmitz, 2015).

Much of the LGBT aging research has not examined the unique needs of transgender elders. Older transgender adults face many unique biomedical and psychosocial challenges. As with older LGB adults, many older transgender adults have faced violence, invisibility, discrimination, and oppression throughout their lifetimes. However, older transgender adults also have faced issues associated with being gender variant in a culture that rigidly adheres to a gender binary. This creates many biopsychosocial barriers for older transgender adults, particularly in accessing health and mental health care as well as social supports and services. For example, transitioning later in life may bring issues around cost, physical dependence, family and relationship dynamics, and end-of-life decisions. For many older transgender adults, facing isolation and poor health outcomes is a reality. A lack of research on older transgender adults leaves gaps in fully understanding these issues and how best to address them (Witten, 2008).

Caregiving and Social Supports

Knowledge about caregiving for older adults in general has increased dramatically in the past several decades. Recently, more research has focused on the caregiving experiences of older LGBT adults, particularly as caregiving occurs in biological and chosen families. While many older LGBT adults benefit from giving care to and receiving care from family members, there are also many challenges associated with caregiving for many in this population. In addition to common challenges that many older adults face in caregiving situations, such as loss of independence and feelings of guilt for being a "burden" on caregivers, some older LGBT adults may also face barriers from health care systems when their families of choice are not recognized as legitimate caregivers (Mayer et al., 2008) and are kept out of decision-making processes. And, estrangement among family members due to older LGBT identities may lead to isolation and barriers for caregiving.

Because of issues with biological family, many older LGBT adults turn to chosen families for caregiving. As with older adults in general, many older LGBT adults report both satisfaction and strain from providing care to a loved one (Muraco & Fredriksen-Goldsen, 2014). However, unlike heterosexual older adults, older LGBT adults may suffer from the erroneous assumptions of others that caregiving does not take a large toll because older LGBT adults are not living "traditional" lifestyles like married or heterosexual older adults (Hash, 2006). These and related issues can lead to additional burdens and barriers for older LGBT adults in caregiving and care receiving, including reduced well-being and increased risk for isolation and institutionalization.

While older LGBT adults are at higher risk than heterosexual older adults for isolation because of barriers surrounding caregiving and other situations, many create sources of social support through friends, partners, neighbors, and families of choice (Orel, 2004), which can improve well-being and serve to protect against poor health and mental health outcomes. Further, older transgender adults may enjoy even larger social networks than their nontransgender counterparts (Cook-Daniels, 2015).

Shifting attitudes about sexual identity suggest that, increasingly, more older gay and lesbian adults will find acceptance from families of origin than gay and lesbian adults from past generations, decreasing stigmatization and internalized homophobia and increasing the strength and number of social supports. This is particularly important for older LGBT adults who may need assistance with finances or caregiving as they age. However, barriers may still exist for older bisexual adults, whose families of origin may question bisexual identities or perpetuate stigma and shame around bisexuality, which still persists in general society (Metlife, 2010).

Older LGBT Veterans and Rural-Dwelling Adults

Aging veterans have specific health and psychosocial needs, particularly older LGBT veterans. Changes to "don't ask, don't tell" and other policy, program, and research initiatives have begun to address the needs of LGBT service members and veterans, including older LGBT veterans. Many older individuals in this population have faced victimization, sexual harassment, sexual assault, and other issues as a result of being a sexual minority in the military. Given the historically hostile military environment for LGBT individuals, older LGBT veterans face increased risk of isolation, homelessness, unemployment, and poor health outcomes when compared to nonsexual minority veterans. Much of this risk comes from reluctance to disclose their sexual identity to health care and other providers in and outside of the veterans service system.

Like older LGBT veterans, older rural-dwelling LGBT adults face unique circumstances and challenges. One in five older adults lives in a rural area (Krout & Hash, 2015), and the composition of older adults increases as the population of a community decreases (Glasgow & Berry, 2013). Populations existing in rural areas are diverse and come with unique characteristics, strengths, and challenges. For example, ethnic minorities accounted for 83% of rural population growth in the decade between 2000 and 2010 (Johnson, 2012), and nearly 15% of same-sex households, representing more than 88,000 families, reside in nonmetropolitan areas in the United States (Grant, 2009; Lee & Quam, 2013).

Challenges faced by those living in older LGBT rural communities include religious and political conservatism (Dillon & Savage, 2006), which can create barriers and challenges for same-sex couples who age in place in rural areas. Further, older LGBT adults face barriers common to all older adults living in rural areas including transportation barriers, income challenges, and a lack of services. Consequently, attending to the needs of and access to resources for older LGBT adults, couples, and families who choose to reside in rural areas is important.

Many older LGBT adults living in rural areas also possess unique strengths that result from living in small, tight-knit communities. Many older individuals and families generally view rural living as safer and healthier than urban living (Watkins & Jacoby, 2007). In addition, older LGBT adults living in rural areas often enjoy more opportunities to develop a sense of community, belonging, and involvement as well as strong social networks than their urban counterparts (Krout, 1988).

Public Policy and Older LGBT Adults

In the past several decades, many policy changes have begun to address the unique needs of older LGBT adults including legislation that has focused on hate crimes, housing discrimination, and marriage and hospital visitation rights. However, a general lack of knowledge of issues facing transgender elders in particular, means rights for this group may not be protected, even with legislation intended to protect these individuals. And, advancing policy and legislation efforts acknowledging and protecting the rights of LGBT individuals have been met with pushback that intends to erode these rights. For example, the Older Americans Act was reauthorized recently, and several provisions for older LGBT adults have been added to the latest version. These provisions seek to bring attention to the unique needs of older LGBT adults and provide support for grants and research to improve services for this population. Sex-reassignment surgeries are now covered by many insurance policies, including those offered through private and governmental entities. And, marriage equality is now a right nationwide. However, many states are responding to these policy changes by enacting legislation that chips away at rights and legalizes the discrimination against LGBT individuals (Fredriksen-Goldsen & Espinoza, 2014).

BEST PRACTICES AND FUTURE DIRECTIONS

Research on issues faced by older LGBT adults has offered helpful guidelines and suggestions for best practices and gaps in many realms that still need to be addressed. Suggestions for future directions in training, services, research, and policy are discussed in what follows.

Training of Professionals and Service Provision

Research on older LGBT adults suggests that more attention needs to be focused on training service providers. Specifically, providers need training around diversity, inclusion, and cultural competence as well as how the intersectionality of age, race, class, gender, sexuality, and cohort characteristics affects older LGBT adults. Providers also need training to develop awareness around the strengths and resiliency of older LGBT adults while attending to common experiences of loss, grief, and bereavement unique to those in this population.

Specific recommendations can be offered for providers to make their practices LGBT- and aging-friendly and affirming. One essential change is to ensure that forms, websites, policies, and other materials used in practice are LGBT inclusive and welcoming. Practitioners can be guided in the use of inclusive language, such as using words like "bisexual" and "transgender" and not using restrictive, binary terms in the forms and materials used in their practices. Practitioners also can be trained to support older LGBT adults they encounter in their practices. This could include recognizing that older adults may experience unsupportive relationships with family, friends, and other providers; being mindful of the historical context and views on homosexuality, bisexuality, and gender nonconformity when older adults were younger and how that history might affect individuals; and recognizing that much depends on when individuals come out as gay, lesbian, bisexual, or transgender and how people might view themselves and the support to which they have access. For example, some older bisexual adults may have difficulties finding community, so providers can recommend online resources for support. Providers could also suggest the use of innovative technologies like telehealth to increase access to services and reduce isolation risk for older LGBT adults who lack social supports or reside in rural areas with few resources. Or, providers could help support organizations and networks that serve the older LGBT community by becoming a referral source for clients, patients, and the community. Much of this training could be accomplished by ensuring providers are trained in and follow competencies developed for professionals who work with this population. And, given low utilization rates of Veterans Health Administration services by older LGBT adults, it is important that community health care providers be adequately prepared and willing to meet the needs of this older population. Providers must be knowledgeable about and sensitive to the unique experiences of older LGBT adults who have served in different military situations and conflicts.

Focus is also needed on improving training of mental health providers to help improve service provision and reduce fear and prejudice among those who provide services. Further, practitioners play an important role in mental health provision for older LGBT adults by addressing heterosexism, acknowledging the role of family and support networks, focusing on historical and social forces that perpetuate oppression, attending to the diversity of older LGBT adults, and focusing on stress as well as resiliency of older LGBT adults (Fredriksen-Goldsen et al., 2014).

Another important recommendation for providers who work with older LGBT adults is the use of models and frameworks that emphasize the intersectionality of factors that contribute to older adults' experiences and that focus on strengths and reduce the use of stigmatizing, pathology-based labels and conceptualizations of issues faced by those in this community. For example, gay affirmative therapy (Harrison, 2000; Van Den Bergh & Crisp, 2004) is one approach that can be utilized to help support older LGBT adults who may struggle with mental health issues. Further, the Minority Stress Model (Meyer, 2003) is a good lens from which to view issues of older LGBT adults, particularly as it relates to experiences of stigma, trauma, violence, and discrimination.

Future Research and Policy Change

Attention has been given to the health, mental health, and long-term care needs and social supports of older LGBT adults in the literature. For example, publications by the Institute of Medicine, *Clinical Gerontologist*, *Journal of Gerontological Social Work*, Registered Nurses Association of Ontario, and *Journal of Homosexuality* have helped to increase the professional attention given to the experiences of community-dwelling older LGBT adults who need home care or assistance in daily living because of health issues. This research has helped to focus on best practices for older LGBT adults including attending to the risk of isolation as well as working with existing strengths such as resiliency and many older adults' ability to form strong social networks.

Future directions in research include increased funding for studies that focus on the intersection of various factors such as age, race, ethnicity, geography, socioeconomic status, and gender and sexual identity to more effectively address health, mental health, and service needs of older LGBT adults. Efforts are needed to conduct research with larger, more diverse sample sizes that result in more descriptive demographic data. This includes the use of innovative sampling strategies that capture subgroups of older LGBT individuals. Further, the continued use of qualitative methods is needed to better understand the unique needs, strengths, and challenges subgroups of older LGBT adults may face around support, self-perception, and service needs and barriers. For example, more research is needed that focuses specifically on older transgender populations, examining the biomedical, psychological, and socioeconomic aspects of aging for this group. Similarly, research is needed to better understand the dynamics of families for subgroups within the older LGBT population, particularly their unique interactions with adult children and grandchildren.

Attention is needed to the diversity existing in rural areas to increase inclusiveness of LGBT elders in research and rural programming and policy considerations. This includes improving the training of social workers who serve rural communities to become more knowledgeable about and sensitive to the needs, desires, and issues faced by older LGBT adults. Social workers could ensure culturally competent service provision in these communities and help older LGBT individuals and families build supportive networks within their towns, which helps reduce isolation and discrimination and increases the safety and visibility of older LGBT adults in these rural communities. Increasingly, organizations like Services and Advocacy for GLBT Elders are helping to reach and serve older LGBT communities, and efforts are needed to continue building and sustaining these supports and networks.

Public policy initiatives and increased funding for these initiatives are vital to promote health and mental health among LGBT elders. Utilizing equity frameworks that focus attention on policy, education, and leadership can address gaps for older LGBT adults with regard to health care and community-based services. Equity frameworks articulate six indicators of access to care for older LGBT adults: environment; community engagement; education and training; programs and services; policies; and leadership. These indicators can assist policy makers and organizations in identifying areas in need of development and changing policies and practices that create service inaccessibilty for older LGBT adults.

Other policy areas affecting older LGBT adults have seen advances, but there is still much work to be done. For example, though the *Outing Age 2010* (Grant, 2009) publication has brought attention to the service needs of older LGBT adults, several recommendations made by the report still need to be carried out, including increased research on the needs of older LGBT adults, the passage of the Equality Act to fight discrimination against LGBT individuals, and increased services to address social isolation of older LGBT adults. And, although same-sex marriage is now legal in the United States and in many other countries, there has been great backlash against the civil rights of these couples as well as all LGBT individuals. There is still much work to be done that not only sheds light on the struggles faced by older LGBT adults, but also that works to effectively end discrimination and brings equity to access to rights and services.

FINAL THOUGHTS

The chapters in this volume highlight the urgency and importance of continuing to work on improving the lives of older LGBT adults through practice, research, and policy. This work is not only crucial for the well-being of the current cohort of older LGBT adults but also for future generations. Continuing this work also honors and builds on the successes and hard work of previous generations of LGBT adults and their allies. It is through their courageous efforts as well as the efforts and voices of allies that attention has focused on the health and well-being of older LGBT adults and changes have occurred in the many institutions and environments with which older LGBT adults interact. Continuing this work means that additional and significant structural and cultural changes can and will occur, chipping away at the institutional discrimination and oppression that contribute to disparities in health, mental health, and social support that so many older LGBT adults have experienced and, ultimately, creating equality for everyone in older age. One respondent from a gay and lesbian caregiving study by Hash (2006) expanded upon the image of what equal rights will mean for same-sex partners:

> Equal rights in the hospital . . . in insurances . . . health benefits . . . and I want to be able to hold her hand in public like husbands and wives do and people who love each other do. I think we have to continue to work towards that. (p. 134)

REFERENCES

Bowleg, L. (2012). The problem with the phrase women and minorities: Intersectionality-an important theoretical framework for public health. *American Journal of Public Health, 102*(7), 1267–1273.

Chiplin, A. J., Jr., Chin, N., Dayton, K., Redman, D., & McIntyre, G. A. (2011). Older lesbian, gay, bisexual, and transgender individuals face special challenges in economic security and health care. *Clearinghouse Review: Journal of Poverty Law and Policy*, 44, 564–577.

Cook-Daniels, L. (2015). Transgender aging: What practitioners should know. In N. Orel & C. Fruhauf (Eds.), *The lives of LGBT older adults: Understanding challenges and resilience* (pp. 193–215). Washington, DC: American Psychological Association.

Dillon, M., & Savage, S. (2006). *Values and religion in rural America: Attitudes toward abortion and same-sex relations.* Carsey Institute, Issue Brief, no. 1. Retrieved from http://scholars.unh.edu/carsey/12

Fredriksen-Goldsen, K. I., & Espinoza, R. (2014). Time for transformation: Public policy must change to achieve health equity for LGBT older adults. *Generations, 38*(4), 97–106.

Fredriksen-Goldsen, K. I., Hoy-Ellis, C. P., Goldsen, J., Emlet, C. A., & Hooyman N. R. (2014). Creating a vision for the future: Key competencies and strategies for culturally competent practice with lesbian, gay, bisexual, and transgender (LGBT) older adults in the health and human services, *Journal of Gerontological Social Work*, 57(2–4), 80–107.

Fredriksen-Goldsen, K. I., Kim, H., Shiu, C., Goldsen, J., & Emlet, C. A. (2015). Successful aging among LGBT older adults: Physical and mental health-related quality of life by age group. *The Gerontologist, 55*(1), 154–168.

Glasgow, N., & Berry, E. H. (2013). Introduction to rural aging in twenty-first century America. In N. Glasgow & E. H. Berry (Eds.), *Rural aging in 21st century America* (pp. 1–13). New York, NY: Springer Publishing.

Grant, J. M. (2009). *Outing age 2010: Public policy issues affecting gay, lesbian, bisexual, and transgender elders.* Washington, DC: Policy Institute, National Gay and Lesbian Task Force.

Harrison, N. (2000). Gay affirmative therapy: A critical analysis of the literature. *British Journal of Guidance and Counseling*, *28*(1), 37–53.

Hash, K. M. (2006). Caregiving and post-caregiving experiences of midlife and older gay men and lesbians. *Journal of Gerontological Social Work, 47*(3/4), 121–138.

Hash, K. M., & Rogers, A. (2013). Clinical practice with older LGBT clients: Overcoming lifelong stigma through strength and resilience. *Clinical Social Work Journal, 41*(3), 249–257.

Institute of Medicine. (2011). *The health of lesbian, gay, bisexual, and transgender people: Building a foundation for better understanding.* Washington, DC: The National Academies Press.

Johnson, K. M. (2012). *Rural demographic change in the new century: Slower growth, increased diversity.* Carsey Institute, Issue Brief, no. 44. Retrieved From http://scholars.unh.edu/carsey/159

King, S. D., & Richardson, V. E. (2015). Influence of income, being partnered/married, resiliency, and discrimination on mental health distress for midlife and older gay men. *Journal of Gay and Lesbian Mental Health, 20*(2), 127–151.

Krout, J. A. (1988). The elderly in rural environments. *Journal of Rural Studies, 4*(2), 103–114.

Krout, J. A., & Hash, K. M. (2015). What is rural? An introduction to aging in rural places. In K. M. Hash, E. Jurkowski, & J. A. Krout (Eds.), *Aging in rural places: Policies, programs, and professional practice* (pp. 3–22). New York, NY: Springer Publishing.

Lee, M. G., & Quam, J. K. (2013). Comparing supports for LGBT aging in rural versus urban areas. *Journal of Gerontological Social Work, 56*(2), 112–126.

Mayer, K. H., Bradford, J. B., Makadon, H. J., Stall, R., Goldhammer, H., & Landers, S. (2008). Sexual and gender minority health: What we know and what needs to be done. *American Journal of Public Health, 98*(6), 989–995.

Metlife. (2010). *Still out, still aging: The MetLife study of lesbian, gay, bisexual, and transgender baby boomers.* New York, NY: Author.

Meyer, I. H. (2003). Prejudice, social stress, and mental health in lesbian, gay, and bisexual populations: Conceptual issues and research evidence. *Psychological Bulletin, 129*(5), 674–697.

Muraco, A., & Fredriksen-Goldsen, K. I. (2014). The highs and lows of caregiving for chronically ill lesbian, gay, and bisexual elders. *Journal of Gerontological Social Work, 57*(2–4), 251–272.

Orel, N. (2004). Gay, lesbian, bisexual elders: Expressed needs and concerns across focus groups. *Journal of Gerontological Social Work, 43*(2–3), 57–77.

Scherrer, K. S., Kazyak, E. A., & Schmitz, R. (2015). Getting 'bi' in the family: Bisexual people's disclosure strategies within the family. *Journal of Marriage and Family, 77*(3), 680–696.

Van Den Bergh, N., & Crisp, C. (2004). Defining culturally competent practice with sexual minorities: Implications for social work education and practice. *Journal of Social Work Education, 40*(2), 221–238.

Watkins, F., & Jacoby, A. (2007). Is the rural idyll bad for your health? Stigma and exclusion in the English countryside. *Health and Place, 13,* 851–864.

Witten, T. M. (2008). Transgender bodies, identities, and healthcare: Effects of perceived and actual violence and abuse. In J. J. Kronenfeld (Ed.), *Research in the sociology of healthcare: Inequalities and disparities in health care and health–Concerns of patients* (Vol. 25, pp. 225–249). Oxford, England: Elsevier JAI.

Witten, T. M., & Eyler, A. E. (2012). Transgender and aging: Beings and becomings. In T. M. Witten & A. E. Eyler (Eds.), *Gay, lesbian, bisexual and transgender aging: Challenges in research, practice and policy* (pp. 187–269). New York, NY: The John Hopkins University Press.

Index

Note: Page references followed by "*f*" and "*t*" denote figures and tables

www.ingramcontent.com/pod-product-compliance
Ingram Content Group UK Ltd.
Pitfield, Milton Keynes, MK11 3LW, UK
UKHW021844100926
8556IPUK00019B/1037

9 780826 125729